Paul Bach-y-Rita (Editor)

Recovery of functic
Theoretical consider
injury rehabilitation

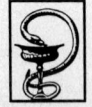

Paul Bach-y-Rita (Editor)

Recovery of function: Theoretical considerations for brain injury rehabilitation

HANS HUBER PUBLISHERS
BERN STUTTGART VIENNA

CIP-Kurztitelaufnahme der Deutschen Bibliothek

Recovery of function: theoretic. considerations
for brain injury rehabilitation / Bach-y-Rita
(ed.). – Bern, Stuttgart, Vienna [Wien]: Huber,
1980.
  ISBN 3-456-80836-4

NE: Bach-y-Rita, Paul [Hrsg.]

© 1980 Hans Huber Publishers Bern
Type-setting by Paul Stegmann Bern
Printed by Lang Druck Ltd. Liebefeld-Bern
Printed in Switzerland

Table of contents

Contributors

PAUL BACH-y-RITA, M.D. Chief, Rehabilitation Medicine Service, Martinez Veterans Administration Hospital, Martinez, California; and Professor, Department of Physical Medicine and Rehabilitation, and Department of Human Physiology, School of Medicine, University of California, Davis

SIMON BRAILOWSKY, M.D. Servicio de Neurofisiología Clínica, Instituto Nacional de Pediatria DIF, and Departmento de Farmacología, Facultad de Medicina, Universidad Nacional Autónoma de México, Mexico D.F.

EDWARD V. EVARTS, M.D. Laboratory of Neurophysiology, National Institute of Mental Health, Bethesda, Maryland

PAUL GLEES, M.D. Anatomy Department, Cambridge University; Professor Emeritus, Institut für Histologie und Neuroanatomie, Universität Göttingen, West Germany

JOSEPHINE C. MOORE, O.T.R., Ph.D. Professor, Anatomy Department, University of South Dakota School of Medicine, Vermillion

MARK R. ROSENZWEIG, Ph.D. Professor, Department of Psychology, University of California, Berkeley

PATRICK D. WALL, Ph.D. Professor, Anatomy Department, University College, London

Preface

Rehabilitation is a new speciality and thus is in the phase of development where most of the procedures used to treat disabilities are empirical. Few procedures have evolved by the logical progression from theoretical concepts and laboratory based research, through clinical research, to accepted therapeutic procedures. This book is a response to the increasing interest in the theoretical bases of therapeutic procedures among rehabilitation professionals.

Each of the authors has a firm grounding in a basic science, as well as an interest in the clinical applications of basic research; each has analyzed and discussed aspects of his field that he or she considers particularly relevant to the development or refinement of therapeutic procedures for brain injured (e. g., stroke and head injury) patients.

The focal point for the preparation of this book was a symposium sponsored jointly by the International Rehabilitation Medicine Association (IRMA) and the Smith-Kettlewell Eye Research Foundation (San Francisco, California). It was held as part of the IRMA III Congress in Basel, Switzerland on July 5, 1978.

The planning of the symposium and the editing of this book were completed while the editor was Professor, Department of Visual Sciences, University of the Pacific and Associate Director, Smith-Kettlewell Institute of Visual Sciences, San Francisco, California.

Particular thanks are due to Dr. Wilhelm Zinn, President of the International Rehabilitation Medicine Association, who was instrumental in the organization of the symposium and in the publication of this book.

Neuroanatomical considerations relating to recovery of function following brain lesions

J. C. MOORE

Introduction

The field of the neurosciences has been and continues to expand rapidly. One can read in the latest research papers, texts or symposia numerous interpretations of how a particular tract, nuclear area, receptor or effector, or a system functions in relation to the external and internal environment. Conjecture, hypothesis, speculation and new concepts are being proposed as never before by researchers and students of the nervous system. In my own studies I have looked at the structure and function of the nervous system (NS) from several different perspectives. (1) Historical data in relation to ideas that were once accepted and later abandoned (or forgotten) and how these beliefs colored our thinking about the NS; (2) Growth and development, i. e., phylogeny, ontogeny, reflexes and/or «genetic memory» and the hierarchy of nervous system functions in relation to archi-paleo-neo concepts; (3) The neurobehavioral sciences in relation to man and other animals; (4) (re)habilitation, especially treatment techniques, neuroplasticity and psychophysiological factors involved in improvement of function following brain injury; and last but not least (5) the ominous trend demonstrated in the last several decades in the way man looks at and attempts to understand the nervous system.

In our teaching, research and clinical practice too much emphasis has been placed upon the structure and function of the phylogenetically newer or more obvious components of the nervous system. The older systems tend to be ignored or forgotten along with the bilateral nature of the nervous system. This trend needs to be reversed. We cannot afford the as-

9

sumption that older structures are unimportant or that they play only minor roles in the integrative nervous system. Every structure has a purpose, in spite of the fact that man has not been able to unravel the mysteries of these structures and relate them to function or loss of function. Those of us who are interested in (re)habilitation need to be aware of all levels and functional interactions of the hierarchical nervous system. We can change these trends if our teaching methods, textbook presentations, research and clinical practice are modified in such a way that we begin to look at each system within the nervous system from a phylogenetic-ontogenetic viewpoint and/or their hierarchical (archi, paleo, neo-) components. We need to understand how each system functions along with all of the other parts of the nervous system. This, on the surface, may appear to be an overwhelming task. In actuality I believe that it is easier to understand the nervous system from this approach than from the classical one. The hierarchical archi-paleo-neo approach helps one appreciate another dimension of neuroplasticity, especially as this relates to (re)habilitation and recovery of function following brain lesion. Granted, there may be an inherent danger in looking at the nervous system from this viewpoint, just as there is when trying to understand it from classical concepts. However, I believe that a greater appreciation and understanding can be gained from this nonclassical approach, especially since it is based upon phylogeny and ontogeny and the integrative action of the nervous system.

This chapter will attempt to look at the N.S. from these perspectives, fully realizing that one cannot cover every aspect of the N.S. in relation to these viewpoints. However, important concepts will be highlighted in order to develop an understanding of the N.S. in relation to neuroplasticity and (re)habilitation.

Historical Data

Man, in his infinite wisdom, has a predilection for dividing the whole up into smaller and smaller parts in order to understand structure and function. In pursuing this bias man learns a great deal about the individual parts, right down to individual cells (GRANIT [23], HORRIDGE [30]). Along with this he establishes a language for communicating information to others and this helps broaden his knowledge about the parts. However, this process, though vitally necessary to gain an in-depth understanding of various structures and functions, can lead to biased thinking. It can actually prevent individuals from looking at the whole in relation to the parts. An excellent example of this fractionation of the nervous system function is found in the man-made divisions of the brain. Long ago certain landmarks were established, based upon embryological research, for demarcating the superior and inferior limits of the medulla, pons and midbrain or various lobes of the cerebral cortex. These «boundaries» have had a tendency to act as fences to the mind, preventing it from gaining a clearer understanding of various parts of the CNS. In actuality no real boundaries exist. Instead there are gradual changes of various structures as the brain stem is ascended from spinal cord levels or descended from diencephalic levels. For example, in the brain stem, the dorsal columns of the spinal cord continue rostally into the lower half of the medulla. The red nucleus of the midbrain extends into the «territory» of the diencephalon. (Some scientists today are even questioning the concept of the «separation» of midbrain structures from the diencephalon and vice versa.) Another example is the vestibular nucleus. This structure overlaps the boundaries «separating» the pons from the medulla. Not only this, but the vestibular nucleus is an integral part, both structurally and functionally, of the juxtarestiform body and the flocculonodular lobe of the cerebellum. The reticular formation, once thought to be limited to the lower pons and medulla, is now known to extend the entire length of the spinal cord, medulla, pons, midbrain, diencephalon and on into the telencephalon (BARR [9], WILLIAMS & WARWICK [54]). When one attempts to understand various functional systems in relation to the entire nervous system, no real boundaries can be found. For example, diseases of the «basal ganglia» or the subcortical nuclear areas of the telencephalon, now include lesions of the red nucleus and substantia nigra of the midbrain, as well as the subthalamus and nuclei of the ventral area of the thalamus, all structures belonging to the diencephalon. When it comes to functional impairment of the vestibular system, a multitude of structures can be implicated extending from the middle and inner ears, the vestibulocochlear nerves, the vestibulocerebellar nuclei and pathways, including the reticular system, the medial longitudinal fasciculus (MLF), the superior cerebellar peduncle, red nucleus and parts of the thalamus, certain components of the visual system including the eyes, and at least two areas of the cerebral cortex, as well as the internal capsule (BARR [9], WILLIAMS & WARWICK [54], PEELE [37]). Many other examples could be cited. The point is, man can no longer be limited in thought by false man-made boundaries. Instead, the entire integrative action of the N.S. must be considered at all levels of the neuraxis. Every part, including all, from the largest to smallest of the interneurons, negative and positive feedback circuits, collaterals and interconnections are vitally necessary for the functional integrity of a normal nervous system. When a part is lost, the functional responsibilities of that area *in relation to all others,* is changed. The resultant sequelle is only a crude outward expression of that for which the nervous system cannot compensate (GRANIT [23], CROSBY, HUMPHREY & LAUER [18], ECCLES [20]).

Another example of fractionation of nervous system functions is found in the cytoarchitectural studies of the cerebral cortex. In the 1800's numerous cortical maps were formulated in an attempt to relate clinical, anatomical, and physiological information to variations in the different developmental and structural layers of the cortex. By the early 1900's BROADMANN's (1909) map or numbering system along with VON ECONOMO & KOSKINAS' (1931) cytoarchitectural maps were widely accepted by the scientific community, along with several other notable contributions. However, few people realize today that most of this interpretive work was done on non-human specimens, yet it was liberally applied to man's cortex (WILLIAM & WARWICK [54], BLAKEMORE [11]). In the early 20th century W. PENFIELD of McGill University published his research concerning stimulation studies of the human cerebral cortex. From this research, generously interpreted by others, the famous motor area 4 (precentral gyrus) and sensory areas 3, 1 and 2 (post central gyrus) plus many others, came into vogue. The findings of BROCCA, WERNICKE and others from earlier research data provided additional information and helped produce cortical maps that were based upon function. To this day these maps are used, almost as gospel, to explain functional localization in the cerebral cortex of man. Yet indepth reading of the historical literature and cross comparisons of different cortical maps including those of HALSTEAD & REITAN, and LURIA'S, leave one puzzled (WILLIAMS & WARWICK [54], BLAKEMORE [11], LURIA [33]). No real agreement can be found among various authors that can substantiate present day concepts concerning discrete functional localization of most of the areas of the cerebral cortex. For one, the depths of the four deepest fissures of man's brain (longitudinal, central (Rolandic), lateral (Sylvian), and calcarine) are relatively inaccessible to stimulation studies, not to mention all of the other sulci of the brain. Buried in these deep fissures lie some of the most important primary receptive/effective centers of the human cortex (Fig.1a, 1b, 1c). Yet most cortical maps locate these areas on the exposed surfaces of the brain. Only a few of the newer maps make an attempt to illustrate some of the various functional areas as we presently understand them (WILLIAMS & WARWICK [54]). Another factor is that it is known that no two brains, or even the two hemispheres of one brain, nor their respective convolutions are alike, except in a very global sense (WILLIAMS & WARWICK [54], ECCLES [20], BLAKEMORE [11], LURIA [33]). In spite of this the old maps persist and perpetuate the myths of the 1800's and early 1900's.

Other factors concerning stimulation studies of the human cortex, and that of feline, canine, simian, etc., need to be considered in light of today's knowledge. The amount, type and duration of the stimulus makes a difference in regard to spread or irradiation effects of the stimulus and the resultant recordings. Every large, small and microscopic part of the brain is now believed to have feedback and feed-forward (ex-

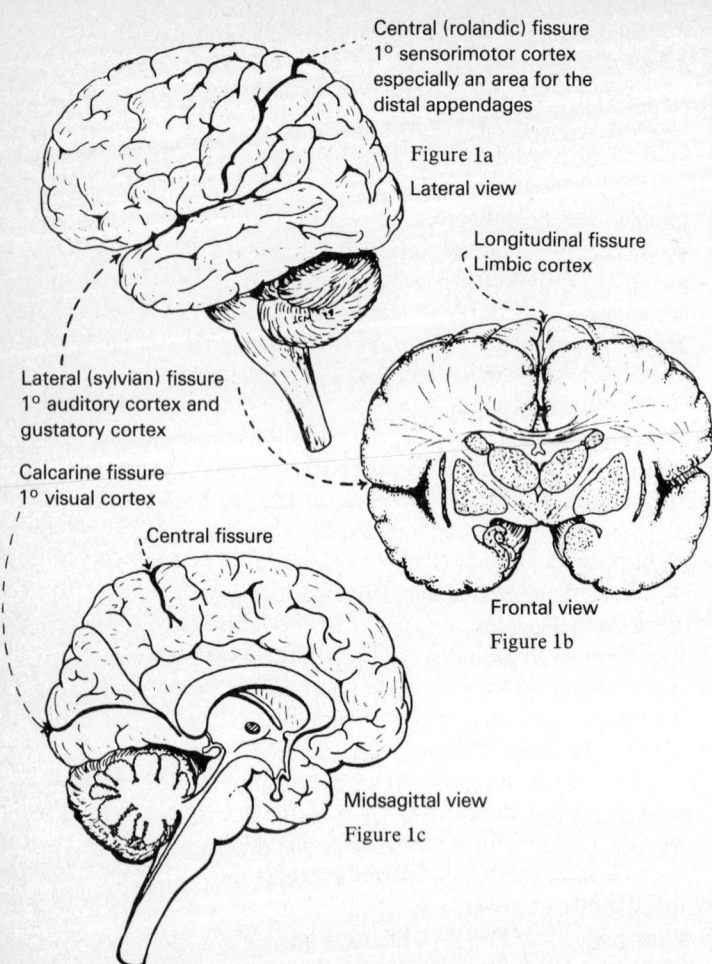

Central (rolandic) fissure
1° sensorimotor cortex
especially an area for the
distal appendages

Figure 1a
Lateral view

Longitudinal fissure
Limbic cortex

Lateral (sylvian) fissure
1° auditory cortex and
gustatory cortex

Calcarine fissure
1° visual cortex

Central fissure

Frontal view
Figure 1b

Midsagittal view
Figure 1c

Figures 1a–c. The deep fissures of the cerebral cortex and the primary functional centers located there in.

citatory and inhibitory) circuitry, not only with adjacent cells, but also with nearby and farther removed nuclear areas, as well as with commissural interneurons and their feedback fibers from contralateral nuclear areas. One wonders what it is that is actually being recorded and interpreted as «function» from these stimulation studies.

Another example is man's fascination for recording information from a single cell in a given area. This is fine, except that it ignores all of the other levels of integrative function associated with the cell that is being probed. Only a small number of articles exist that investigate, simultaneously, all of the various structures concerned, for example, with vision (GRANIT [23]). Along with recording from a cell in the primary visual cortex (Area 17), information should be gathered from the superior colliculi, lateral geniculate nuclei, the pulvinar, and associative visual areas, such as areas 18 and 19 bilaterally, the frontal eye fields (lower area 8) as well as the anteriomedial temporal lobes and inferior parietal-superiolateral temporal lobes, not to mention the cingulate gyrus and the septal area. Even if only four of these areas could be probed simultaneously, we would know a great deal more about the integrative action of the N.S. than merely concentrating on the primary visual cortex or the lateral geniculate nuclei. This entire issue is clouded further by such factors as (1) the level of anesthesia used on the animal before and during the studies and/or the amount of depression of the reticular activating system, an area that is extremely vulnerable to many of the drugs used on research animals; (2) restraints and the position of the animal (side lying, upright, prone, supine, etc.) during the research and the effects of these postures on the vestibuloproprioceptive systems and the resultant recordings; (3) the degree of excitability or fear in the animal before and during the study due to the odors and strangeness of the environment; (4) whether or not light and sound is occluded from the animal and the effects of these stimuli on the function of the brain; and last, but not least (5) the duration of the operative procedure in regard to respiration, postural restraints, metabolism, fluid balance, etc. All of these parameters and more can affect the results of any research and especially one that attempts studies related to the complex interactions of the human nervous system. In my opinion, before man can gain a better understanding of his own nervous system, he has to realize that this system or any part of it does not function in isolation from any other part. Normal function depends upon the integrity of the entire system and the total animal within his normal environment. Therefore, in lesion studies and/or stimulation studies, or any study wherein the animal is anesthetized, confined or in a strange environment the results are a reflection of the compensatory activity of the nervous system at that particular moment in time. The results rarely reflect the normal integrative action of the system. Similarly, what is seen following a lesion in the human nervous system, no matter where it is, may not be a true reflection of the functional capabilities of the remaining structures, or of the area where the lesion occurred (GRANIT [23], CROSBY, HUMPHREY & LAUER [18], ECCLES [20]). Rather, what is examined for sensorially, or is seen motorically, is a reflection of the cumulative reaction of an incomplete and compensating nervous system. The resultant clinical interpretations of the remaining functional capabilities are biased by what can be observed, palpated, or interpreted from multiple clinical tests coupled with the examiner's knowledge of the nervous system. For example, if the examiner has been trained to look at and mainly test the motor side of the N.S. and also thinks of this system in terms of contralateral cortical control via the «pyramidal» and «extrapyramidal» systems, then his mind is pre-set to hear, feel and understand only that which he knows. If he turns to the clinical references for clarification of his beliefs and clinical findings, he will have a tendency to find information that will substantiate his beliefs. At the same time he will have a predilection for ignoring or dismissing that which is conflicting, strange or different. The ultimate expression of this is man's ability to «turn-off» or «tune-out» anything that a patient attempts to relate about his/her abberant perceptions and functional abilities (or inabilities) during the recovery process following nervous system insult. Here, however, is an opportunity for understanding the complex interactions of a malfunctioning system, a system that is trying to recuperate and reorganize itself in relation to what was once a normal system. However, if the reports offered by the patient, concerning aberrant feelings or lack of functional abilities fail to correlate with the rehabilitationists' or researchers' perceptions of how things should be, this valuable and extremely vital information is lost – forever. Very quickly the patient learns what the experts desire to hear, see or feel. This, of course, reinforces and perpetuates established biases and erroneous concepts concerning the N.S.'s ability to reorganize and recover (to some unknown degree) over a prolonged period of time. Similarly, this «tuned-out» atmosphere sets up a climate of sensory deprivation, not only for the expert but more so in regard to the patient and his/her nervous system's potentials. Do we need thousands of written case histories, like those of Dr. A.BRODAL (BRODAL [14]), Dr. P.BACH-y-RITA (BACH-y-RITA [8]), and others, before we are willing to open up the intellectual barriers of our minds and begin to listen? Are thousands of case histories necessary before we are willing to accept and recognize the fascinating potentials that are available within the nervous system for stimulating and enhancing the recovery process through multiple therapeutic techniques, each geared to individual patient needs? Certainly the hundreds, if not thousands, of research articles concerning the effects of sensory deprivation and enriched environments, as well as those dealing with sensory substitution and sensory-integrative techniques, should constitute a reliable basis upon which we can reject the outdated and time-worn classical concepts concerning the structure and function of the nervous system and readily accept new ideas. Once this is accomplished it should open up vast unexplored potentials for (re)habilitation. This should enable clinicians to look upon each patient as a «research model» capable of relaying valuable data concerning loss and recovery of function following N.S. insult.

Phylogenetic and ontogenetic trends in CNS development

Phylogenetically, one of the most primitive forms of life had a diffuse nerve network (Coelenterates). When primitive worms (Convoluta) appeared, this network became organized into groups of cells (or ganglionic masses), the largest of which were concentrated toward the cephalic regions of the

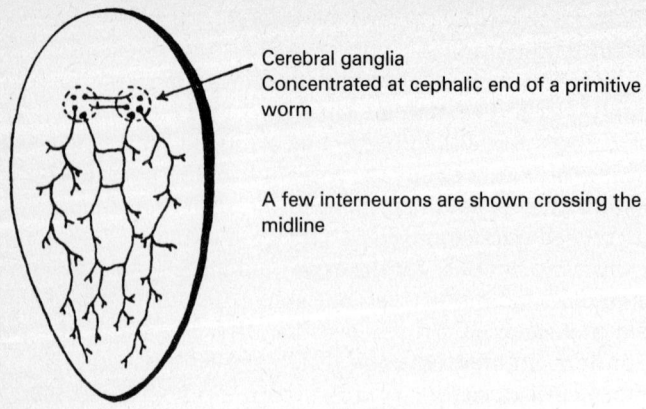

Cerebral ganglia
Concentrated at cephalic end of a primitive worm

A few interneurons are shown crossing the midline

Figure 2. Non-segmental organism with ganglia concentrated and organized at the cephalic end.

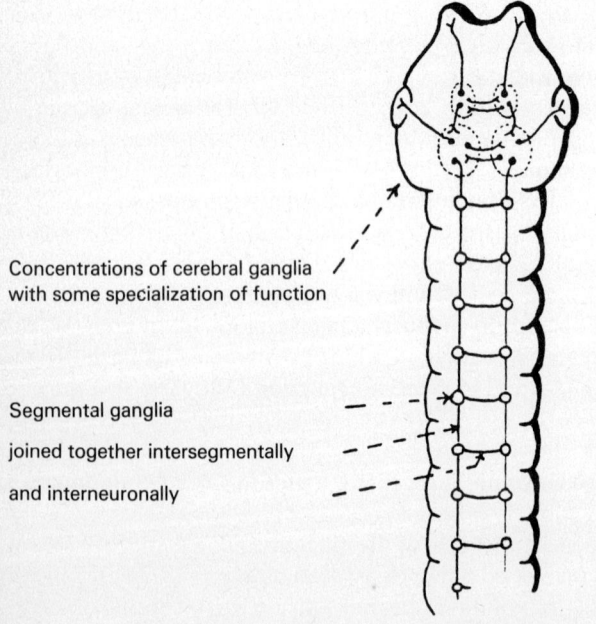

Concentrations of cerebral ganglia with some specialization of function

Segmental ganglia

joined together intersegmentally

and interneuronally

Figure 3. Segmental organism with additional cephalic ganglia and ganglia at each segmental level.

organism (Fig. 2). Segmentation came next. Concentrations of cell bodies (ganglia) were organized at each segmental level, and strung together intersegmentally by neuronal processes. At the rostral end of the organism (Annelids) larger ganglionic masses appeared (Fig. 3). Segmentation, unlike the non-segmental forms of lower invertebrates, became a developmental law in the evolution of vertebrates. This arrangement enabled fractionation of function in relation to sensation and established a trend for the eventual ability of the organism to localize stimuli and respond with primitive protective reflexes/responses. This led to a «division of labor» and/or energy conservation between various sensorimotor components in relation to the external (exteroceptive) en-

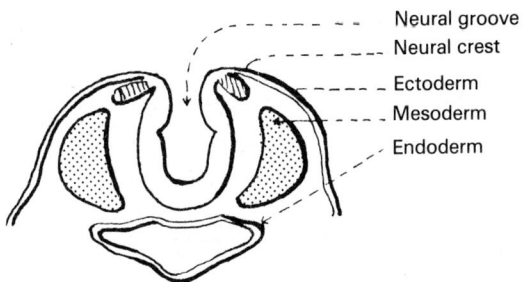

Figure 4a. Neural groove and neural crest stage of the developing embryo. (x-section of dorsal area.)

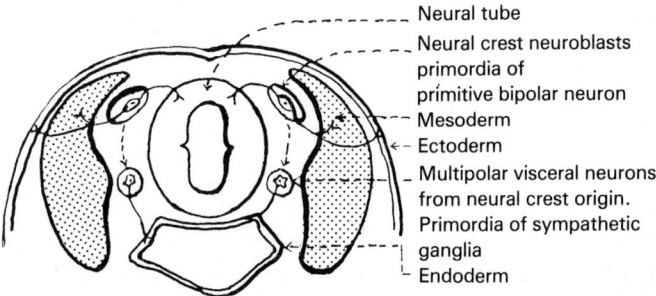

Figure 4b. Neural tube stage showing primordia of sensory neurons of developing embryo. (x-section of dorsal area.)

vironment, proprioceptive systems and the internal (interoceptive) environment. For example, the progenitors of our primary receptor neurons (neuroblasts of neural crest origin (Fig. 4a, 4b), are organized so that the peripheral processes or primitive bipolar neurons are connected with ectodermal segments as well as the mesodermal or segmental myotomes (Fig. 5). Later in evolution these primitive bipolar sensory neurons «specialize», i.e., separate ones develop for perception of exteroceptive stimuli, while others specialize for the reception of proprioceptive stimuli (Fig. 6). (The multipolar cells of neural crest origin continue to function as visceral effectors, i.e., they constitute the general visceral efferent sympathetic

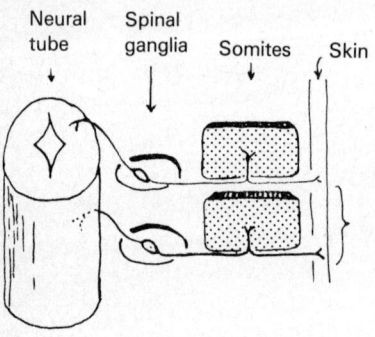

Figure 5. Primitive bipolar sensory neurons supplying ectodermal and mesodermal structures.

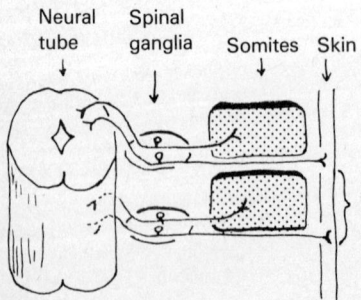

Figure 6. Pseudounipolar sensory neurons specialized for somites and ectoderm.

20

system of the autonomic nervous system (ANS) in higher vertebrates and man (Fig. 4b).) In spite of this division and further specialization of sensory neurons, an intimate functional association remains between ectodermal and mesodermal structures in regard to N.S. function. For example, an adequate stimulus of a dermatomal area associated with the underlying musculature results in a facilatory response in these muscles and a dampening or inhibitory response of their antagonists. This is one of the basic theories used by clinicians to support various treatment techniques used in rehabilitation and/or reflex testing for determining the integrity of normal N.S. function and/or abnormal responses resulting from various lesions. Many additional primitive protective reflexes and/or normal reflexes that appear following CNS insult have their basis in this primitive segmental relationship and the once primitive mutual innervation of exteroceptive and proprioceptive structures (Fig. 5).

Cell bodies of multipolar motoneurons of the developing neural tube remain in the basal plate (Fig. 7). Only their axonal processes follow the migration of the dorsal and ventral myotomes that will eventually cover all areas of the body. Throughout vertebrate phylogeny, the motor components undergo relatively minor changes in comparison to the sensory systems. These systems are the ones that become of ma-

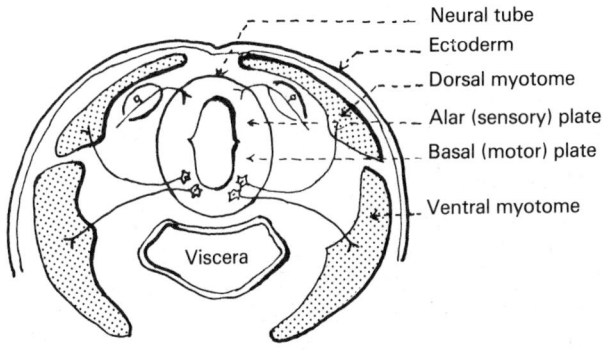

Figure 7. Multipolar motoneurons supplying the dorsal and ventral myotomes in the developing embryo.

jor importance throughout evolution, especially in regard to nervous system development, cephalization, maturation and function. The motor systems remain as «servants» to the rest of the N.S., i.e., they can only respond or not respond, depending upon the integrity of the sensory systems coupled with the integrative action of the nervous system (TUCHMANN-DUPLESSIS, AUROUX & HAEGEL [50]).

In primitive vertebrates the bipolar sensory neurons synapse directly upon the ventral multipolar motoneurons, enabling the organism to reflexively move, or freeze, in response to stimuli. This constitutes the primitive simple reflex arc (Fig. 8). In man, the only remnant of this is the myotatic (stretch) reflex (Achilles tendon reflex or patellar tendon re-

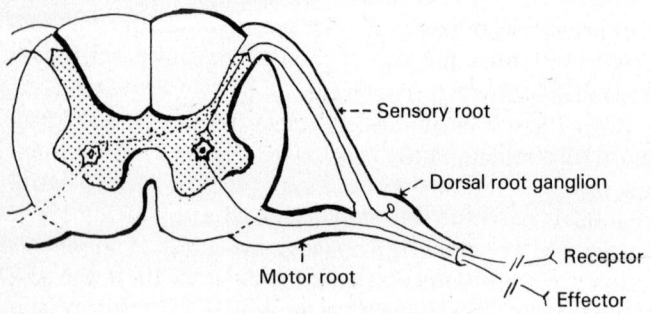

Figure 8. The primitive «simple» reflex arc or myotatic (stretch) reflex.

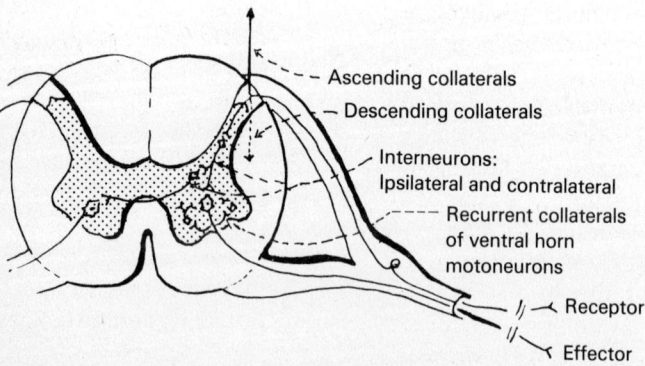

Figure 9. The «complex» reflex arc with collateral fibers and interneurons.

flex), that helps sense muscle length, velocity, tension, extension and/or muscle tone. All other reflex/responses are much more complex, i.e., at least three neurons are involved, including important feedback circuits, ascending and descending collaterals and extremely important commissural interneuronal connections (Fig. 9). In man, the majority of the reflex/responses depend upon complex circuitry that evolved in the higher vertebrates, and especially in mammals, over eons of time. No longer can we attempt to explain reflexes on a simple sensory to motor sequence. Instead, one must keep in mind the fact that thousands of neurons and their terminal processes are involved in regulating the threshold of a single cell body in any given location in the CNS, just as one single cell within the CNS can influence or synapse upon hundreds or thousands of other neurons (GRANIT [23], BARR [9], WILLIAMS & WARWICK [54], CROSBY, HUMPHREY & LAUER [18], ECCLES [20]). (Within the cerebellum, one neuron can have as many as 100000 synapses impinging upon its dendritic processes.) Likewise, when attempting to understand normal and abnormal movement or lack of movement, one must consider all of the sensory receptors and CNS pathways involved in detecting and perfecting a movement and/or a postural change and not just the motorical components that produced the movement. (See section on receptors involved in movement.)

In summary, seven major and consistent trends are found throughout the evolution of the nervous system. (1) The migration and formation of groups of cell bodies into ganglionic masses along the neuraxis along with the development of synapses. (2) Larger concentrations of ganglionic clusters at the rostral end of the organism, i.e., cephalization. (3) Segmentation and fractionation of function in respect to reception and localization of stimuli. (4) Preservation of the phylogenetic relationship between ectodermal receptors and the muscle or myotomes. (5) Continued specialization and importance of sensory systems in comparison to the motor systems. (6) The development of complex reflex and feedback circuits, collateralization of neurons and the multiplicity of synapses impinging upon each neuron in the CNS. (7) The development of the interneuron. These major phylogenetic trends constitute the foundation upon which one can gain a better understanding of nervous system function, plasticity and recovery. Several of these trends will be discussed in greater depth in order to relate phylogeny with the structure and function of man's nervous system.

Development of the interneuron

Modification of sensorimotor reflexes, integration and coordination of function within the organism evolved with the development of interneurons. By definition, interneuronal cell bodies and their processes are confined within the CNS. Decussating interneurons first appeared in the rostral areas of the CNS of lower vertebrates (Amblystoma). These intercalated neurons functioned as connecting links between the multisynaptic ascending «sensory» pathways and the multisynaptic descending «motor» pathways (Fig. 10). With the development of this type of interneuron, total body reflex movements, away from the side of the stimulus, evolved. Later in evolution, commissural interneurons developed at all levels of the neuraxis (Fig. 9). This change enabled the organism to modify total body reflexes in favor of segmental reflex control especially in response to stimuli impinging upon different segments of the body. This was the beginning of fractionation of movement in response to various stimuli as well as being the progenitor of future genetic (or pre-programmed) reflex potentials that would be «laid-down» in man's N. S. Examples of these are the withdrawal (nociceptive) reflex, primitive rooting, sucking and swallowing reflexes, swimming and grasping reflexes, placing, stepping, crawling, cruising and walking reflexes, the Landau and Babinski reflexes, symmetrical and asymmetrical tonic neck reflexes, etc.

As the evolutionary trend toward cephalization progressed – several other types of interneurons developed other than commissural interneurons. Some interneurons did not cross over to the contralateral side of the neuraxis. Instead they re-

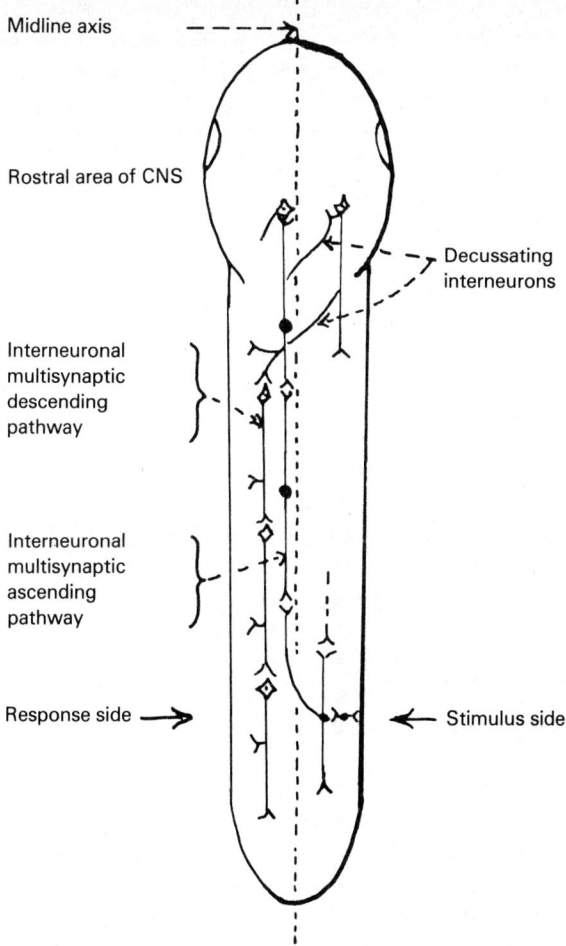

Figure 10. Primitive interneuronal systems of a hypothetical organism.

mained ipsilaterally and became intercalated between primary sensory, or receptor neurons, and motor neurons (Fig. 9). Others developed in very specific areas of the gray matter. Examples of these would be «Renshaw cells» and other small interneurons in the ventral horn gray that are part of the excitatory or inhibitory feedback circuits affecting α, β, and γ motoneurons (Fig. 9). Still others became interposed between descending «motor» pathways and the final common pathway of lower motor neurons. Some remained in the dorsal gray horn (alar plate) in areas like substantia gelatinosa and nucleus proprious (Rexed's lamina II–IV). These small interneurons may serve as «immediate feedback circuits» for dampening or enhancing certain kinds of sensory input along with supraspinal pathways that synapse upon these interneurons to help modify incoming sensory information (WILLIAMS & WARWICK [54]).

Longer interneurons, classically referred to as second order or third order (secondary or tertiary) neurons of ascending pathways, and «extrapyramidal» and «pyramidal» tract neurons of the descending pathways, gradually appeared throughout evolution. Almost all of the ascending and descending fibers constituting the white matter of man's CNS are interneurons. Few, if any should be called 2°, 3° neurons, or pyramidal tract neurons, or whatever classical name is applied. There are several reasons for this. (1) Many second order neurons are actually third or fourth order neurons. (2) The majority of the so-called «pyramidal tract» fibers are interneurons consisting of various sizes, lengths, and conduction velocities, the majority of which synapse upon other interneurons before synapsing on α and γ motoneurons. Similarly, few of the «pyramidal» fibers are involved in the control or regulation of motoneurons. Instead, many influence centers that are concerned with modifying incoming sensory information, and/or relaying information to subcortical nuclear areas, including the cerebellum. (3) The old use of classically named pathways carried with it the connotation that ascending pathways are «sensory» while the descending ones are «motor». In actuality, they are neither sensory nor motor, i.e., they are integrative and act in this capacity at all levels of the neuraxis. (4) These classical tracts are still thought of as if they were rather «clean and pure», i.e., a tract begins in one nuclear area and ascends (or descends) without collateralizing, to another nuclear area. Quite the contrary. Most pathways, with the exception perhaps, of the very recent phylogenetic tracts, have numerous collaterals projecting into adjacent nuclear areas of the neuroaxis through which they pass. (5) The newer pathways that may not have collaterals may compensate for this lack by having multiple paralleling fibers that (a) originate in the same area; (b) carry similar coded messages as the «parent» non-collateralized fiber; and (c) accompany the main fiber for various distances along the neuraxis before synapsing in nuclear centers along the way. In this manner, different levels of the neuraxis are continually informed, both ipsilaterally and contralaterally (via commissural interneurons) concerning that which is important to the total system at any given moment. (6) These interneurons do not carry «pain», «touch», «proprioceptive» or «motor» kinds of information. Instead they transmit a coded message that is modified or changed at every synapse. Many incoming coded messages never get beyond the first or second synapse, i. e., the input is inhibited especially if the information is not critical at the moment or is «already known» by the organism. Coded messages that are transmitted beyond the first synapse are continually modified at each successive synapse by the circumstances of the moment, the immediate future, and the past, or the organisms' genetic heritage coupled with learned and/or environmental experiences that have been incorporated into its nervous system.

Today, it would be wise to abandon the classical concepts attributed to the ascending and descending pathways and begin to think of these as interneuronal systems. Once this is accomplished the integrative actions of the nervous system, along with the concept of polysensory neurons and the bilateral nature of the nervous system can be understood, especially as these relate to neuroplasticity.

The bilateral nervous system

Phylogenetically a major function of commissural interneurons is to transmit information occurring on the ipsilateral side to the contralateral side of the nervous system and vice versa. These interneurons form commissures at *all levels* of the neuraxis. The preponderance of these fibers cannot be ignored, as they are responsible for the bilateral coordination of the nervous system and of the entire body. It is interesting to note that commissural interneurons do not decrease in number as the phylogenetic scale is ascended along with increasing cephalization. Rather, there is an increase of commissural neurons, of which the corpus callosum is the largest and best known. In spite of this, the functional importance of commissural interneurons has been ignored in favor of overemphasizing the phylogenetically recent crossed pathways and hemispheric specialization of cortical areas in relation to the «laterality» of man's nervous system. Granted, man uses one limb more precisely than the other for some specific functions, such as writing, and perhaps eating, and reaching for objects. But few individuals can get dressed, take part in sports, be musicians, painters or clinicians without utilizing the entire body in the activity. Everything man does on one side of the body immediately affects and is affected in turn by the opposite side. SHERRINGTON called our attention to reciprocal innervation and crossed extensor (or flexor) reflexes (double reciprocal innervation), as did CAJAL, ECCLES, GRANIT, and many others (GRANIT [23], ECCLES [20], BLAKEMORE [11], SHERRINGTON [47]). They recognized the bilaterality of the nervous system and the tremendous importance that this has in relation to normal function. In spite of this, emphasis is placed upon lateralization of function. Perhaps this evolved from clinical studies and man's tendency to understand that which can be seen, palpated, or readily tested, i.e., the obvious, or the gross motor deficit that appears on one side of the body following brain injury on the contralateral side (Ref.: BRODAL [14], CHUSID [16]). The individual who has never experienced hemiparesis fails to see or recognize the subtle changes and deficits that occur on the ipsilateral side. This bias is reflected in our terminology, i.e., hemiplegia (or hemiparesis), hemianopsia, hemiballism, alternating or crossed hemiplegia, etc. These terms and many others imply «laterality», i.e., only one side of the body or a part is affected. In reality, both sides are affected – one side being much more involved and the other to some lesser degree. But this «lesser degree» is such that the «good side» fails to function normally (BRODAL [14]). How can this be explained? Basically, the more involved side has lost its ability to send normal coded messages concerning events occurring on that side, to the opposite side, via the commissural interneurons. Similarly the involved side is no longer capable of receiving normal coded messages from the contralateral side. Another way of expressing this would be that the less involved side experiences sensory deprivation. Not only is it unable to handle the aberrant signals constantly received from the more involved side, but it is deprived of receiving normal integrative input from all levels of the neuraxis, and especially from various nuclear centers that send their fibers both ipsilaterally and contralaterally, i.e., bilaterally, up and down the neuraxis. To explain. If one looks in greater depth at the com-

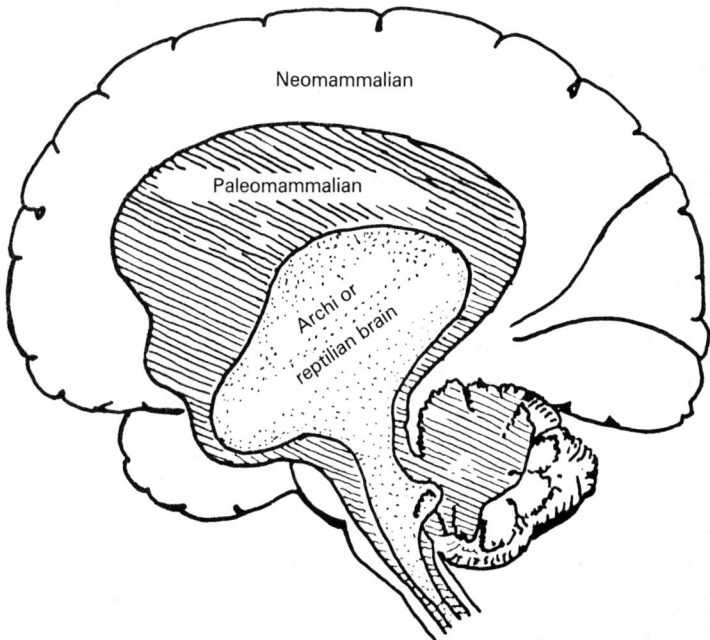

Figure 11. The archi, paleo, and neo parts of the mammalian central nervous system.

plex structure and function of the CNS an interesting evolutionary pattern develops that gives credence to the bilateral nature of man's nervous system. Phylogenetically and ontogenetically the nervous system develops in a hierarchical sequence. The oldest or archi systems are the first to develop and function, followed by the intermediate or paleo systems. Last to appear are the most recent or neo systems. At birth, the archi systems are functional, as are some of the paleo or protopathic systems. However, many of the neo or epicritic systems do not obtain full functional capabilities until years after birth. There are numerous examples of these three systems that can be cited. For instance, the entire CNS can be

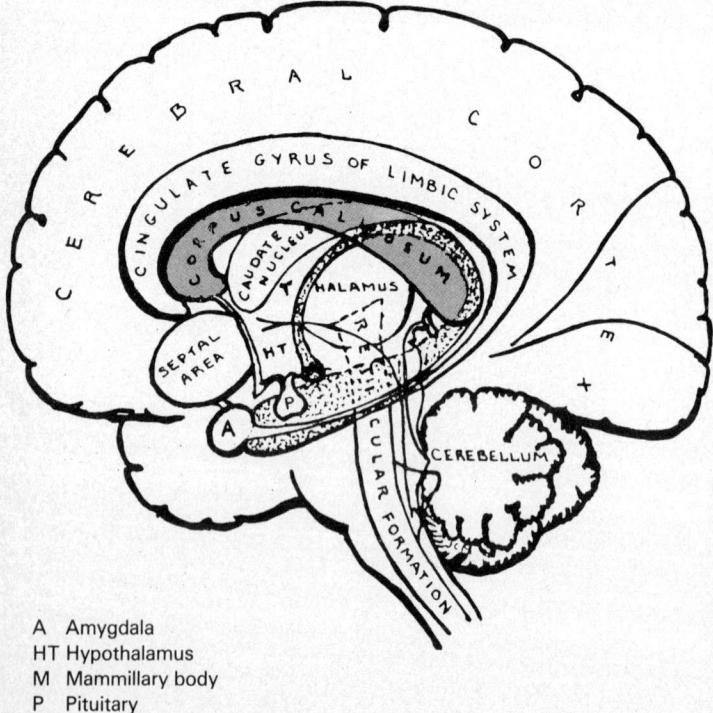

A   Amygdala
HT Hypothalamus
M   Mammillary body
P   Pituitary
▨   Hippocampal-fornix system

Figure 12. (Correlate with Fig. 10.) Some of the major components of the archi, paleo, and neo structures of the mammalian central nervous system.

«divided» into the archi or reptilian CNS, the paleomammalian part and the neomammalian CNS (Fig. 11, 12). The reptilian component is the central core of man's CNS, or the autonomic nervous and reticular systems of the neuraxis, and the archicerebello-vestibular system. The paleomammalian part constitutes the protopathic or protective systems, while the neomammalian represents the epicritic or exploratory components of the CNS (Figs. 11, 12, 13). It is interesting to note that the majority of the neuronal processes projecting from nuclear centers of the archi systems do so bilaterally. Also, these fiber systems are highly multisynaptic in character (Fig. 14). The pathways of the paleomammalian system tend

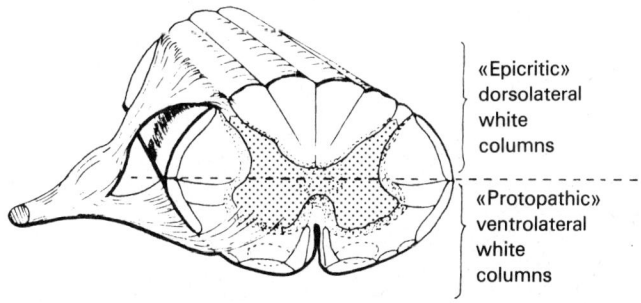

«Epicritic» dorsolateral white columns

«Protopathic» ventrolateral white columns

Phylogenetic concept re development and function of the spinal cord

Reticular and ANS pathways / Central gray of spinal cord	Oldest or archi and the first to myelinate and function.
Ventrolateral white columns	Intermediate or paleo in age and believed to myelinate and function next i.e. protopathic or protective. More concerned with primitive reponses and gross patterns of behavior.
Dorsolateral white columns	Most recent or neo and last of spinal cord pathways to myelinate and function, i.e. epicritic or exploratory. More concerned with learned behavior.

Figure 13. The archi, paleo, and neo components of the mammalian spinal cord.

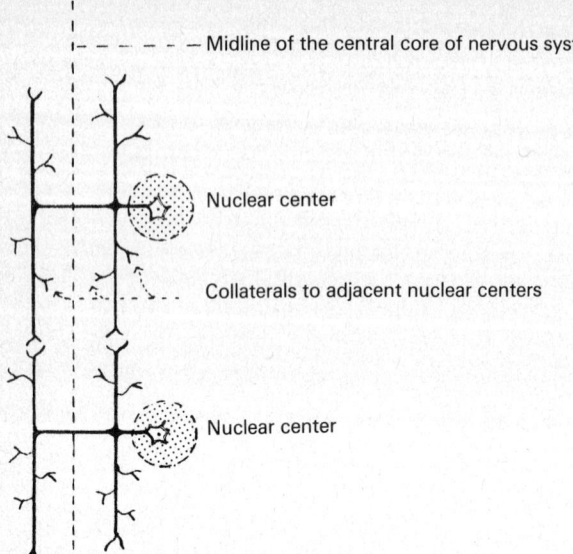

Figure 14. Archi-types of CNS neurons with bilateral ascending and descending neurons and numerous collaterals to adjacent nuclear centers. Schematic.

to decussate and exert their major influences contralaterally, but also they usually have minor, though important ipsilateral components. These systems also have fewer multisynaptic connections in comparison to the archi systems (Fig. 15). The neo-cerebral systems appear to give man «laterality», i.e., these nuclear centers and the fibers projecting from them are principally involved in influencing the contralateral side of the body while the neo-cerebellar systems principally influence the ipsilateral side. Also, these neo-pathways have the most direct fiber systems between lower and higher centers or vice versa (Fig. 16). It cannot be forgotten, however, that all three of these systems (archi, paleo, and neo) along with their respective nuclear centers and fiber projections, synapse with commissural interneurons. Thus the bilaterality of the nervous system is preserved in spite of the evolutionary trend toward «lateralization» of function.

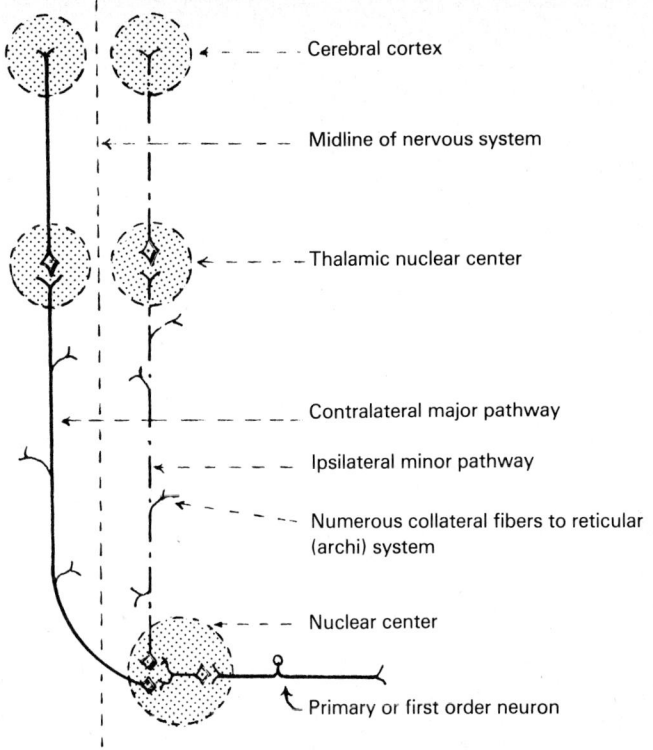

Figure 15. Paleo-type of ascending CNS neurons with major contralateral and minor ipsilateral tracts. (Descending paleo-pathways have similar configurations.)

Another important aspect of the «bilateral» nature of the nervous system could be termed spatiotemporal «stereomorphophysiology», i.e., the study of structure and function of an organism in relation to three-dimensional time and space. Orientation in space, both in relation to oneself as well as the environment is a critical factor, not only for survival but for moving, exploring and learning from one's internal and external environment. Man has long recognized that the structural and functional components of our visual system endows us with stereoscopic vision. Likewise, the shape of man's (or animal's) ear (pinna), as well as all of the components of the

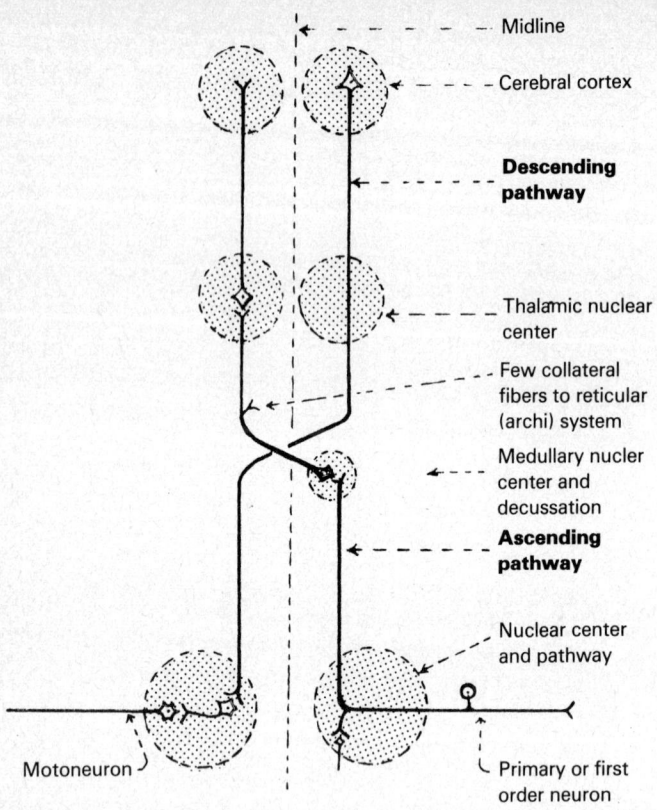

Figure 16. Neo-types of CNS neurons with major contralateral pathways. Schematic.

auditory system, including the contralateral, ipsilateral and commissural connections, enables us to have stereophonics, or a three-dimensional perception of sound. This ability is continually utilized for auditory spatiotemporal orientation, as well as for understanding language, music, etc. An indepth study of the structure and function of the vestibular system, i.e., the semicircular canals, ducts and their respective receptors including their ipsilateral, contralateral and commissural fibers, enables man to have stereoequilibrium, or spatiotemporal orientation in all three planes of movement. The gravitational receptors (graviceptors) of the vestibule of the labyrinth (maculae sacculae and utriclae) and their component pathways endows us with «stereograviorientation», because of the three dimensional characteristics of these receptors in relation to the three planes or forces of movement in respect to gravity. The special senses of smell and taste, like the visual, auditory and vestibular systems, have bilateral structural and functional components and commissural systems that endow us with «stereo-olfaction» and «stereogustation». In other words, the special senses, with their predominately bilateral receptors, bilateral pathways and commissural fibers enables the body to orient its «three dimensional self» into three dimensional time and space, – something that would be impossible in a nervous system that lacked bilateral receptors, pathways and commissural fiber systems.

Are these «stereomorphophysiological» characteristics limited to the special senses, or can the same or similar stereo-abilities be found within the receptors, pathways and effectors of the general sensorimotor systems? The answer is obvious. Almost all of our receptors, including the general graviceptors, found in joint capsules, tendons, muscles, fasciae, in and around internal organs and in the skin (epidermis and dermis) enables man, both subcortically and cortically to have spatiotemporal or stereogravitational as well as stereognostic capabilities. Therefore, we know consciously and especially subconsciously, where we are in space, both in respect to our body parts relating to the whole organism, and the whole in relation to the surrounding environment. Likewise, in handling or manipulating objects, our stereognostic abilities enables us to perceive three-dimensional multisensory information about objects that we choose to examine, use as tools, or use for something new. Rarely does our nervous system allow us to examine a new object that is totally unfamiliar to us, with one hand. Rather, like infants and children, we examine it bimanually and stereoscopically. We may even express new thoughts or ideas out loud and assume «questioning postures» or express inner feelings with body language gestures, while attempting to ascertain what it is that we are examining. All of this bilateral or stereomultisensory input from the entire body, coupled with re-afferent (feedback) from our motorical expressions and behavioral mannerisms, enables us to gain a better three-dimensional understanding of the object in respect to its shape, weight, texture, coolness or warmth, color, «feeling», moveable parts, etc. This behavior also helps in our attempt to identify and/or relate it to something that we already know. In other words, we tend to revert to bilateral exploratory behavioral patterns that are similar to and are readily observable in the developing infant and child, i.e., during the time when our immature nervous systems were becoming familiar with our own bodies as well as exploring and learning from the stereo-environment. Practically everything that man (or animal) does, (work, play, or activities of daily living), is accomplished by the bilateral, three-dimensionally organized and integrative nervous system. This endows man with highly refined stereocapabilities and enables us to relate to and survive in our three-dimensional environment.

Fortunately, a vast amount of this stereoability is integrated in the nervous system at subcortical levels. The phylogenetically older levels of the system continually set and reset the necessary background chemical, emotional and muscular tone, including coordination, balance and timing that is necessary for normal stereofunctioning, learning, and manipulating the three-dimensional environment.

It is only in the neo-evolutionary systems of higher primates and man's nervous system that one finds a trend away from bilaterality and towards a degree of laterality or specialization of hemispheric function. This in no way negates the subcortical or lower level bilateral organization of the stereo systems. Instead, this reinforces them. Not only are the subcortical systems, both structurally and functionally, the foundations upon which the neo-systems function, but the neo-components, via the corpus callosum and lesser known commissures of the diencephalon and midbrain, add a new stereo-dimension to the nervous system. This endows man with an ability to have knowledge about the environment, adapt to it, and communicate this knowledge in various ways to offspring as well as future generations. The asymetrical cerebral hemispheres also appear to be specialized, not only for storage and retrieval of basic knowledge (or the ability to learn, adapt and act consciously and purposely), but for the ability to have an added three-dimensional cognition of the environment in an almost unlimited spatiotemporal sense. This also endows man with adaptability potentials that are far and beyond those of most other animals in the environment. Similarly this enables man to have the capabilities of manipulating and changing the environment, not only in our own territory but into that which extends beyond the horizon. At the same time man can adapt to immediate needs, or future ones, depending upon the seasons, the food supply and the demands of each individual and the group or society to which he belongs.

In summary, man's two hemispheres appear to be specialized for different degrees of awareness and storage of information about himself and the environment. However, the two sides readily share their receptive, cognitive and expressive abilities, via commissural connections, in order to achieve a gestalt-like perception and appreciation of the total environment, including every facet of its parts. This functional specialization endows man with a vastly increased storage capacity for knowledge of the past, functioning in the present and anticipating the future. It heightens his abilities to consciously perceive and express himself in a multi-adaptable and multi-talented manner in order to survive in a multidimensional world.

Trauma to the CNS destroys, to a greater or lesser degree, the three-dimensional or stereomorphophysiological nature of the system. Unfortunately, the phylogenetically newer components are usually more severely involved in comparison to the older parts. For one, the neo structures and functions are more vulnerable because (1) their metabolic demands are much greater in comparison to older components; (2) their blood supply is not as well established, i.e., the neo systems are usually less vascularized than the older ones; and (3) they are structurally more susceptible in that they are located on the surface or near the periphery of the CNS. Another reason is that the neo-systems are extremely dependent upon the older components of the nervous system for setting the background tone or postural adjustment, timing and co-ordination of stereotyped patterns of movement. Likewise, the reverse of this is that the older systems, in order to carry out these functions, are dependent upon certain inputs from the neocortex and neocerebellum for inhibiting «unnecessary» activity in the older subcortical systems including areas in the brain stem and spinal cord. This is so, not only in a gross functional sense but also at the microscopic level in relation to regulating the delicate facilatory and inhibitory balance of thresholds of billions of individual cells at all levels of the neuraxis. This enables the phylogenetically newest components of the neo systems to carry out higher cortical functions without having to expend excess energy regulating and coordinating the lower systems. Trauma, of course, changes these parameters (BRODAL [14]). Not only are the subcortical regulatory mechanisms released from cortical inhibition, but these lower centers lose some or most of their ability to regulate and establish the necessary foundation upon which the higher centers are dependent for normal function. Concurrently, the bilateral three dimensional nature of the system is interrupted. The involved area loses the ability to receive normal input, via commissural fibers from the «non-involved» side, as the «non-involved» side is deprived of normal input from the contralateral areas effected by the lesion. The remaining subcortical, and especially the neo-cortical centers, once so dependent upon lower areas for normal function and vice versa, have to expend excess energies, not only in interpreting a multitude of aberrant signals, but just as important, a *deficit* of signals upon which it was once totally dependent.

In summary, any lesion of the CNS results in a diminution of the bilateral nature of the N.S., i.e., both sides of the organism are affected in a structural and functional sense. This in turn diminishes the ability of the organism to relate to its three dimensional self and the environment. It stands to reason that the greater degree of severity of the brain lesion, the greater is the loss of function on the opposite side of the body, because of the vulnerability of the neocortical systems and because these are predominately crossed systems. However, this loss is reflected on the ipsilateral side due to extensive interruptions of commissural fiber systems, as well as association and projection fibers that enable the body to function as a bilaterally integrated whole. The fact that man fails to recognize the subtle (and sometimes not so subtle) changes that occur on the «good side» following a lesion, does not negate the fact that there is a greater or lesser diminution of normal function and perception, especially in relation to sensorimotor stereotyped patterns of movement and semi-automatic learned reflexes on the «non-involved side». Perhaps, when this is recognized and accepted as fact, then many of our rehabilitation principles will be better understood and especially those that are founded upon the knowledge of developmental sequences, spatiotemporal adaptation, and principles concerning the subcortical sensorimotor integrative action of the nervous system.

The importance of cervical levels of the neuraxis

In the embryonic development of man and higher vertebrates, two major systems begin developing and functioning in the first three weeks of life. The cardiovascular system is first, followed very closely in time by the development of the primitive nervous system. The cardiovascular system matures rapidly unlike the nervous system that takes up to two decades, or longer, before it reaches full functional and emotional maturity (ECCLES [20], MOORE [35], LEMIRE, LOESER, LEECH & ALVORD [31], MOORE [34]). Initially, the neural tube begins closing at cervical levels of the spinal cord. With additional maturation, tubal closure continues cephalically at a slightly faster rate than caudally. From this basic developmental pattern the cephalocaudal law of development was established. However, if one correlates phylogenetic developmental patterns with embryonic development along with the onset of function, the cephalocaudal law, per se, needs to be modified. Instead, the law should be restated as the *cervico*cephalocaudal law of development (Fig. 17). Placing em-

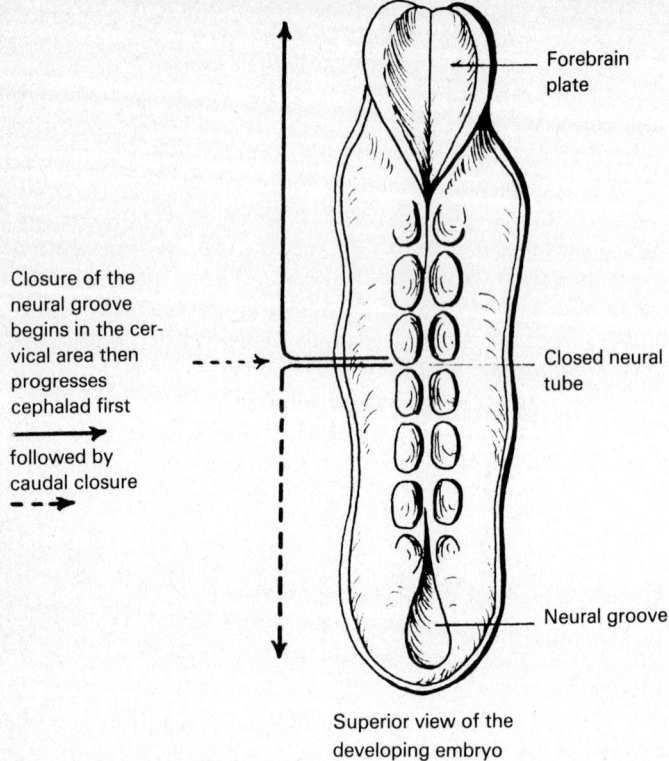

Closure of the neural groove begins in the cervical area then progresses cephalad first

→

followed by caudal closure

- - →

Forebrain plate

Closed neural tube

Neural groove

Superior view of the developing embryo

Figure 17. The «cervicocephalocaudal» law of development as seen in the developing embryo.

phasis upon the cervical levels in regard to growth, development, balance, coordination and function establishes the importance of this area of the nervous system and the body, especially in relation to (re)habilitation. For example, it is almost impossible for all other systems of the nervous system to function normally when there is a lack of stability, coordination and purposeful movement patterns, including normal feedback information, at the cervical level of the body. This area is the key point for controlling the head and the rest of the body in relation to the head. It is interesting to note that just as the nervous system begins developing here, the mature

Chart A. The major ascending and descending pathways of the central nervous system from spinal cord levels.

	Cervical levels	High thoracic	Thoracic levels	Lumbosacral levels

Ascending pathways — Originate at levels indicated

	Cervical levels	High thoracic	Thoracic levels	Lumbosacral levels
1. Fasciculus gracilis ⎫ Dorsal column pathway			▓	▓
2. Fasciculus cuneatus ⎭	▓	▓		
3. Lateral spinothalamic tr.	▓	▓	▓	▓
4. Ventrospinothalamic tr.	▓	▓	▓	▓
5. Dorsal spinocerebellar tr.	▓	▓	▓	
6. Ventral spinocerebellar tr.				▓
7. Cuneocerebellar tr.	▓	▓		
8. Spino-olivary tr.	▓			
9. Spinotectal tr.	▓			
10. Spinoreticular tracts.	▓	▓	▓	▓

Descending pathways — Terminate at levels indicated

	Cervical levels	High thoracic	Thoracic levels	Lumbosacral levels
11. Lateral corticospinal tr.	55%	20%	23%	
12. Ventral corticospinal tr.	▓	▓		
13. Rubrospinal tr.	▓	?	?	
14. Tectospinal tr.	▓	▓		
15. Tegmentospinal tr.	▓	▓		
16. Lateral vestibulospinal tr.	▓	▓	▓	▓
17. Medial vestibulospinal tr. (of MLF)	▓	▓		
18. Medial longitudional fasc. (MLF)	▓	▓		
19. Olivospinal tr. (?)	▓			
20. Reticulospinal trs.: A.N.S. part and to α and γ motoneurons		SNS	P SNS	
	▓	▓	▓	▓

41

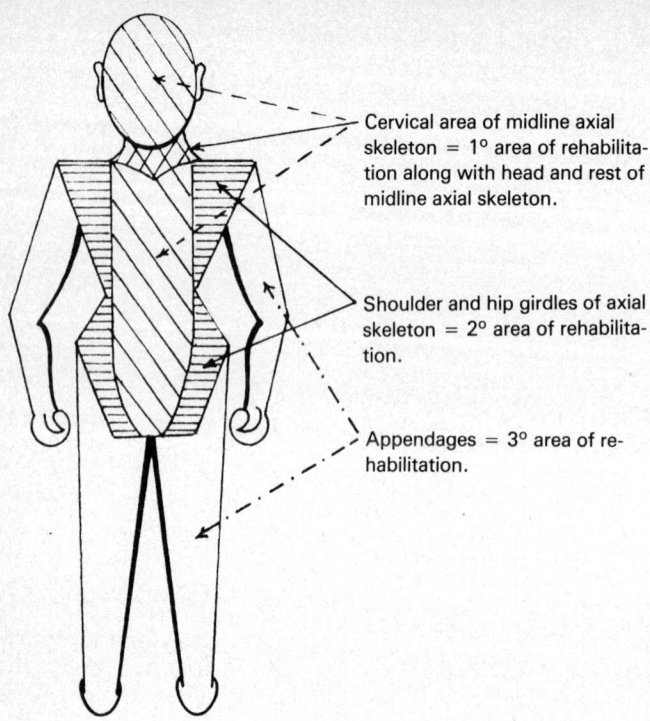

Cervical area of midline axial skeleton = 1° area of rehabilitation along with head and rest of midline axial skeleton.

Shoulder and hip girdles of axial skeleton = 2° area of rehabilitation.

Appendages = 3° area of rehabilitation.

Figure 18. The cardinal areas of the body in relation to rehabilitation principles.

nervous system also expresses, both structurally and functionally, the importance of this area. For example the majority of ascending or descending pathways begin or end here. Even the crossed component of the «pyramidal» tracts or lateral corticospinal tract (of those fibers destined to reach spinal cord levels) sends 55% of its fibers to cervical levels, while only 20% continue on to thoracic levels and 25% to lumbosacral levels (BARR [9]). Granted, a large component of these fibers, destined for cervical levels, are necessary for upper limb functions, but many are for afferent and efferent regulation of neurons that «fine tune» the neck musculature. The small uncrossed component of the «pyramidal» tract (ventral corticospinal tracts) sends almost all of its fibers to this level, the rest going to highest thoracic levels. Other pathways, either ascending or descending are noted in Chart A. Similarly, many of the critical reflex/responses of the body originate at cervical levels before «spreading» up, down and across the system to affect the rest of the organism. The tonic neck reflexes and labyrinthine (vestibular) reflexes (also known as the postural and righting reflexes), may act initially at cervical levels. Visual reflexes to peripheral stimuli and auditory reflexes to sound are mediated via tectospinal, tecto-reticulospinal, and tegmentospinal tracts to cervical levels (ABRAHAMS [1], ABRAHAMS, RICHMOND & ROSE [3], ABRAHAMS [4], ABRAHAMS, RANCIER & ROSE [2]). The chain reflexes or body-on-body reflexes, as well as most of the primitive avoidance reflexes all manifest themselves in movement, initially at cervical levels. Suffice it to say that the cervical levels of the neuraxis are critical, and must be considered as a primary area for restoration of function following nervous system insult.

If indeed our present concepts concerning (re)habilitation are correct, then the cervical levels and associated pathways, along with phylogenetically older receptor-effector systems should be considered as one of the corner stones of the (re)habilitation process (Fig. 18). Lack of stability at cervical levels results in decreased stability in the rest of the trunk, as well as the shoulder and hip girdles. Instability in these areas is irradiated into the appendages, including the head, and especially into the distal parts of the limbs. Conversely, distal instability, if that is the area primarily affected, creates proximal and midline instability. Unless the distal part can be stabilized, in some manner, so that the midline area can function normally, this area cannot pre-set the necessary background muscle tone, coordination and patterning needed for guiding proximal and distal limb movement. Whichever is the case, a vicious cycle results. Instability in the appendages, along with lack of head control, sets up a multitude of aberrant feedback signals, especially from the visual, vestibular and other proprioceptive systems that are attempting to coordinate head-neck and body movement. Not only this, but aberrant signals are constantly being received from the body's extero-proprioceptive systems, and especially from those areas that are the most severely affected. The damaged CNS is incapable of handling these aberrant inputs. In attempting to cope with these extraneous messages, the CNS dampens or inhibits movement in order to eliminate, as much as possible, all of the aberrant stimuli that it is receiving. In so doing, it is able to achieve a greater degree of midline stability. This in turn allows the organism better utilization of the special senses (visual, auditory and gravivestibular) so that it can achieve a more normalized relationship with itself in respect to the environment. Case in point. Many «athetoid» cerebral palsied children develop into «tension athetoids» as they mature into adulthood. Individuals with spasticity and ataxia gradually become less mobile and more rigid in their movement patterns, as they mature. The adult hemiplegic, and those with Parkinsonism, multiple sclerosis, combined systems disease, etc. exhibit increasing paucity and/or rigidity of movement as their disease process progresses. The same can be seen in *normal* individuals as they progress through life. Is this decline in mobility *always* the result of nervous system deterioration or pathology, or is it, *in part,* a reflection of an adaptation process that is present at all ages and stages of life? In other words, is this, in part, an adaptive survival mechanism that enables the organism to cope with the environment and itself during times of stress, disease or injury? This process automatically helps inhibit undesirable aberrant input and allows the organism to cope more effectively until it recovers. For example, a «stiff neck» or «low back pain» immediately sets up a total body pattern that has the necessary degree of immobility in order to gain midline stability and diminish undesirable input from the area sending pain signals. Should the pain continue for an extended period of time, the body assumes an acquired semi-rigid posture in an attempt to adapt to the most comfortable and least mobile position.

Pain is used here as an example because everyone is familiar with the effects that this has upon the system in respect to decreased mobility and/or paucity of movement. Also this demonstrates an inherent adaptive process of how the nervous system copes with undesirable stimuli. Few of us have

44

perceived the kinds of aberrant signals, such as loss of verticality, apraxia, astereognosis, agnosia, hypesthesia, hyperreflexia, hemiplegia, etc., that the brain-injured individual experiences. Yet we have all seen and worked with people whose nervous systems are constantly bombarded by aberrant sensory perceptions and abnormal movement patterns. Where appropriate therapeutic intervention is lacking, we have witnessed how instability patterns and aberrant stimuli can subtly create, over an extended period of time, a gradual lessening of distal and proximal mobility that eventually results in an almost rigid stabilization pattern of the body's midline structures. Yet these midline areas, and especially the cervical levels must have *stability coupled with free flowing patterns of midline mobility* (i.e., trunk rotation and lateral bending combined with flexion/extension patterns) in order for the organism to optimally utilize its general, and especially, its special senses for orientation in space and survival. Stability is the foundation upon which normal patterns of mobility develop (GRADY, GILFOYLE & MOORE, to be published [22]). Midline stability, coupled with mobility, becomes the foundation upon which proximal and distal movement patterns develop, including the necessary feedback stimuli from these areas into the midline structures, which reinforces midline-stability-mobility patterns (GRADY, GILFOYLE & MOORE, to be published [22]). In the brain-injured these vital stability-mobility patterns and servomechanisms are affected. Man and other animals are subcortically dependent upon these midline structures for automatic regulation of muscle tone, synergy, timing, balance and subtle postural adjustment and for coordinated patterns of movement of the entire body. Without them, the animal cannot survive. Man does, as long as he can be cared for by others.

In the brain injured we not only see a disorganization of normal stability-mobility patterns and aberrant feedback information, we see a nervous system that is adapting to these extraneous movements and faulty perceptions by inhibiting mobility while attempting to gain stability. If the system is allowed, or allows itself, to carry this adaptive process to extremes, then paucity of movement resembling total body rigidity can result. If this process continues, the sequelae may be disuse atrophy, «frozen» joints and sensory deprivation, all of which enhance the deterioration of the organism. Much of this syndrome can be prevented, either by therapeutic invention or by the organism's own attempt to rehabilitate itself. I am reminded of the elderly father of a friend of mine who had a severe CVA and became «paralyzed» on one side of his body. Upon «recovering» he was sent home to his cabin in the north woods of Michigan to «live out his days» as a bed-ridden cripple. This former woodsman refused to give up. When spring came, he literally crawled out of bed on hands and knees and managed to reach his garden. Day after day he worked the soil and eventually planted his garden, on his hands and knees. Throughout the summer he continued this activity while cultivating and harvesting. During the long winter and into the seasons that followed he carried on similar activities until he was able to function almost normally. Several years of «all fours» crawling, leading to knee standing, cruising and eventually standing and walking activities enabled him to rehabilitate himself. Little did he know that he was «instinctively» following the phylogenetic and ontogenetic growth and development patterns akin to those he had used subcortically when he was an infant, toddler and young child. He was unconsciously reestablishing the balance and integrity of older midline structures of the neuromuscular system before attempting to regain functional integration in the newer centers. By supporting himself on his hands and knees and sometimes on his elbows, in order to use his hands, he dampened out abnormal distal movements and hence faulty feedback signals, in favor of gross bilateral stability-mobility patterns. He had automatically forced himself (and his nervous system) to reestablish head-neck control along with bilateral midline trunk and proximal limb girdle stability-mobility by adopting the all-fours position, and then moving within the limits of this pattern. This also forced his body to work rhythmically and symmetrically and precluded the possibility of substituting maladaptive behavioral patterns. Fractionation and smoothness of patterned movements came in gradually as his system regained sufficient bilateral trunk stability *and* mobility. Only at this time did he begin to work towards the upright position, but only after regaining sufficient balance, strength and coordinated control of his body axis and proximal limb girdles. He eventually became self-sufficient. He spent the rest of his life providing for his needs by chopping wood, gardening, trapping and caring for himself.

Is there scientific research supporting rehabilitation concepts that state that there is a need to reestablish symmetrical midline stability and mobility before attempting to rehabilitate the more distal parts of the body? Is there evidence that supports the use of the cervicocephalocaudal law of development and/or the use of developmental sequences as a valid therapeutic technique? Or more specifically, are any of the therapeutic techniques used today in (re)-habilitation supported by hard scientific data? Certainly one case of a northwoodsman rehabilitating himself by instinctively following certain rehabilitation principles does not give credence to these concepts. However, I believe that the structure and function of the nervous system, as we know it today, does offer scientific evidence to answer these questions and many more. Nature is conservative (GRANIT [23]). She has experimented, over eons of time, with this structure we call the nervous system. The hierarchical developmental sequence of this system (phylogenetically and ontogenetically), is well documented. The manner in which various systems and their neuronal connections begin to express themselves behaviorally is well known and this should constitute reliable evidence upon which scientific facts can be found to support certain (re)habilitation principles based upon these developmental sequences. We know which systems must develop first and begin to function before other systems can express themselves (LEMIRE, LOESER, LEECH & ALVORD [31], PEIPER [38]). It is also known, that, in individuals with brain lesions, one usually sees a loss of hierarchical systems in a reverse structural and functional sequence. The neo-components are usually the most vulnerable to trauma and are the last to recover, if at all. They appear to be less plastic in that they are principally «lateralized». Neofunctions such as fine manipulative hand movements, communication skills, higher forms of learning, memory, judgement, emotional control and «intelligence», are believed to be hemispherically localized (DIMOND & BLIZARD [19]). The phylogenetically older systems, which appear to be more plastic, are endowed with a greater number of polysensory synaptic connections, feedback circuits, commissural fibers and genetic memory or pre-programmed reflex/responses. Also they are more bilaterally organized and redundant (GRANIT [23], ECCLES [20]). Their major role is that of regulating cell body thresholds for maintaining the basic needs of the organism so that it can survive. It is through these phylogenetically older systems that the newest components express themselves and upon which they are totally dependent for their functional integrity.

In the majority of brain-injured individuals, no matter where the lesion occurs, the functional interaction and dependency of the neosystems upon the older ones is disrupted. Lower and older subcortical centers of control are released from higher inhibitory influences just as the higher centers no longer receive a balanced integrated input from the lower centers. Likewise, the areas of the body that are utilized for controlling and fine tuning our movement patterns and are responsible for higher cortical functions such as reading, writing, speaking and skilled manipulations, are usually the most severely affected. It is interesting to note in this regard that the smallest muscles of the body are primarily the ones that endow man with the abilities noted above. It is also noteworthy to mention that the majority of these small delicate muscles are endowed with the highest muscle spindle population densities. Similarly, practically all of the muscles in our body that have the highest spindle densities, in comparison to the mass of the extrafusal muscles, are found in those structures that are critical to the functional integrity of the neo-systems, or those qualities that make man uniquely human. The intrinsic muscles of the hands, richly endowed with muscle spindles (including their CNS connections), gives man his writing skills and fine manipulative abilities. The extraocular eye muscles enables animals to scan, track and fixate on objects, but more so, they play an important role in the fine saccadic movements that man uses for reading, writing, painting, or performing delicately guided manual skills. The intrinsics of the larynx aid in speech modulation, as the intrinsics of the middle ear muscles help us fine tune that which we hear. The muscles of facial expression endow man with extremely subtle gradations of movement for non-verbal communication skills. Last, but not least, are the vast number of small muscles of the vertebral column and especially those of the cervical areas. These are richly endowed with muscle spindles and control extremely fine head movements as well as setting the background for a multitude of fine postural adjustments for the rest of the body (RICHMOND & ABRAHAMS [42], RICHMOND & ABRAHAMS [43]).

One dare not disregard the anatomy of the nervous system or the neuromusculoskeletal system and say that structure does not necessarily imply function or recovery of function following CNS insult. Detailed knowledge of neuroanatomical structure, embryology, growth and developmental sequences and comparative anatomy has been known for decades. Unfortunately, in many cases this information has not been integrated into our knowledge because the functional implications that this data provided, especially in regard to (re)habilitation, eluded man. However, this does not give us license to continue to ignore the fact that the hierarchical and redundant structure of the nervous system is «trying to tell us something» (GRANIT [23]).

In summary, the cervical area of the body appears to be the pivotal point upon which many of man's gross and fine sensorimotor functions depend. Lack of bilateral stability and mobility in this area is irradiated into the trunk and limbs. Instability along with aberrant feedback is usually manifested by cervical immobility, resulting from the nervous system's attempt to dampen or inhibit abnormal movement in order to gain some degree of meaningful control over the body. The special senses, located in the head, are dependent upon the cervical areas of the spinal cord and vertebral column for their functional integrity. In light of this, the cephalocaudal law of development should be reevaluated in accordance with the neuroanatomical structural and functional importance of the cervical levels of the neuraxis. Perhaps restating it as the cervicocephalocaudal law of development and function would be more appropriate, especially when this concerns (re)habilitation of brain injured individuals.

Sensory systems

Classically, the general sensory components of the nervous system are presented, and remembered, as rather «pure» inputs. For example, pain and temperature (coolness and warmth) travels via the lateral spinothalamic pathways, or touch (crude or gross tactile), pressure, vibratory and proprioceptive or position sense, or tactile (fine discriminative or two-point tactile) senses and their respective pathways are all taught as rather basic structural and functional components of the nervous system. Also, these senses are utilized in clinical testing and research as almost pure forms of input. The special senses, auditory, visual, vestibular and gravireceptors, and taste and smell, are also taught and/or tested as if they were «pure inputs». However, the nervous system does not function in response to «pure» data input. Instead, it is constantly being bombarded by a multitude of highly variable stimuli. A parallelism could be drawn between this «multisensory» input and a thousand-piece orchestra. The kettle drums, violas, violins and bassoons, along with the piccolos, drums, the harp and the horns are all engaged, at various moments, in creating a continuum of beautiful music. Likewise, each instrument, of and by itself, is producing individual notes of continually varying intensities and tones and blending these notes in with entire composition. Does the listener hear the single A-string of the violin or the C-note of the french horn and state that these instruments are critical to the functional integrity of the orchestra, or does he hear the entire ensemble? The answer is obvious. However, man has a tendency to look at the orchestration of the nervous system only in respect to the violin and the french horn, or perhaps the kettle drum. He fails to acknowledge the whole orchestration. Part of the reason for this is the way in which he was trained. The other reason may be due to a lack of understanding of the complexity of «multisensory» inputs in relation to the hierarchical structure and function of the nervous system. In other words, one must understand, at least conceptually, all of the instruments in the orchestra, not only in relation to where each instrument is located in respect to every other instrument, but also in relation to the total orchestra and the surrounding environment. Also, each instrument must be understood in relation to its own individual structure, variability, intensity, and range, and the kind of notes it can produce at any given moment, and when it is supposed to sound forth so that it will be in harmony with adjacent instruments and the entire ensemble. This example conceptualizes the orchestration of the multisensory nature of the afferent and reafferent (sensory feedback) components of the nervous system. It also enables one to recognize that practically every sense or stimulus known (or yet to be discovered) is continually sending or not sending some kind of coded message into the CNS at any given moment. These signals are finely tuned or graded, i.e., they are extremely variable, depending upon the internal and external environmental demands of the system. Similarly, these coded messages and their effects upon the system depend in part upon the degree of maturity of the system, including its genetico-environmental heritage, and the immediate and long term future of the organism. With such a complexity of messages continually bombarding the system, the organism must have a means whereby it can (1) conserve energy, both structurally and functionally in order to meet the demands of the environment; (2) be able to send or not send an appropriate stimulus complex of messages at any given moment; and (3) be able to handle this information when it reaches the CNS.

Does conservation of energy support the classical Doctrine of Receptor Specificity? If this doctrine stands, it would imply that the nervous system would have to consist of an infinite variety and unlimited number of receptors in order to orchestrate all of the subtle gradations of stimuli constantly being received by the CNS. Likewise, trillions of cell bodies would be needed in every part of the CNS to properly handle this input. But every nervous system appears to have a finite number of receptors and CNS neurons (GRANIT [23], BARR [9], CROSBY, HUMPHREY & LAUER [18], ECCLES [20], SHERRINGTON [47]). Nature, over eons of time, has «experimented» with different modes of transmission of impulses, various types of receptors and a variety of nervous systems. In so doing she has been able to utilize different receptors and cells within the nuclear centers of the CNS with a multiplicity of functions. For example, the Pacinian corpuscle and its component fiber was once thought to be a pressure receptor. Research indicates that it is also an excellent vibratory receptor, as well as a gravireceptor. Under extreme conditions, it may be able to transmit «pain». It is also susceptible to extreme changes in temperature, i.e., it changes its signal frequencies under these conditions (WILLIAM & WARWICK [54], SATO [46]). The neuromuscular spindle is capable of registering a variety of functions such as muscle length, velocity, tension, and static (tonic) and kinetic (dynamic) position sense. Research has indicated that it may be sensitive to pressure (WILLIAMS & WARWICK [54], BRIDGEMAN & ELDRED [13], WILLIS & GROSSMAN [55]). It is an excellent vibratory receptor (WILLIAMS & WARWICK [54], ARUTIUNIAN [7], BROWN, ENGBERG & MATTHEWS [15], TROTT [49], WILLIS & GROSSMAN [55]). Like the Pacinian corpuscle, it may be capable of transmitting a type of «pain» signal under certain conditions, and it appears to respond differently with temperature changes (WILLIAMS & WARWICK [54], URBSCHEIT & BISHOP [51]). The receptors of the labyrinth are no longer believed to be limited in their functions to the detection of gravity, rotatory and linear movement, including changes in acceleration and deceleration. They are also known to be sensitive to certain flutter and vibratory frequencies and pressure changes (BARR [9], WILLIAMS & WARWICK [54], SARNAT & NETSKY [45], WILLIS & GROSSMAN [55]). Many other examples could be cited, including a number of receptors (Ruffini end organs, Golgi-Mazzoni receptors, tactile disks, some forms of bulbous corpuscles, and a variety of joint receptors) whose multitude of functions are either unknown or highly controversial (WILLIAMS & WARWICK [54], WILLIS & GROSSMAN [55]). Perhaps this controversy stems from the fact that under varying conditions a given receptor can react to different kinds of stimuli, instead of being limited to just one, two, or three kinds as was previously believed. In other words, each receptor may have an optimal threshold for the reception of a particular type of stimulus at a given moment, but by changing the internal and external parameters of the organism, a receptor can react to, and transmit information from, a broad spectrum of stimuli. This would be more consistent with the phylogenetic studies that show how various types of receptors utilized by invertebrates for survival, have been modified and carried over into vertebrate evolution, and again modified as the phylogenetic scale is ascended to man (SARNAT & NETSKY [45]). In spite of these changes, many of man's receptors are very similar, both structurally and functionally, to those found in invertebrates and lower vertebrate forms of life (SARNAT & NETSKY [45]). In other words, it would appear that throughout evolution nature has utilized a finite number of receptors and has «endowed» each kind with the capacity to receive a variety of stimuli, depending upon the circumstances. For example, there are a great number of different kinds of receptors in our bodies that are capable of registering vibratory stimuli in the 50 to 250 (or 300) Hz range and higher (WILLIAMS & WARWICK [54]), WILLIS & GROSSMAN [55]). Likewise, there are a vast array of receptors that register flutter stimuli (1 to 50 Hz range) (WILLIAMS & WARWICK [54], WILLIS & GROSSMAN [55]). Instead of evolving specialized receptors for each of these frequencies, nature has been conservative and has enabled receptors that respond to other types of stimuli (such as pressure, muscle length, touch, tactile, proprioception and auditory input) capable of responding to a variety of frequencies. Other examples could be cited. Suffice it to state that we should begin to think in terms of multipotential receptors, just as we are accepting the theory of polysensory neurons in the CNS.

Along with the concept of multipotential receptors is that of the total organism being involved in all patterns of movement. No part of the body works in isolation from any other part. The slightest change in posture and/or movement in one area calls for total body readjustments in all other segments. This activity is registered immediately in various nuclear centers of the CNS. This information is compared or matched against total body data compiled from the previous position, the input from the change that is taking place, and the results of the change in respect to the next moment in time, coupled with the entire pattern of activity that is yet to be completed. As each movement is successfully accomplished and repeated over and over, the total movement pattern is refined and smoothed out (BOWER [12]). Timing sequences are perfected along with the right degree of muscle tone and synergy of stability and mobility. Any activity that is being perfected, or has been in the past, is continually analyzed, refined and re-monitored by the vast array of receptors that are feeding information into the integrative nervous system. For example, the visual system via cranial nerves II, III, IV, VI, along with the cervical cord levels, and perhaps V, (including the para-sympathetic component of III and the sympathetic nervous system component, functioning together in control of the in-trinsic eye muscles, for light, accomodation and vergence re-flexes), are sending in signals relating to the surrounding en-vironment as well as those parts of the body that lie within its peripheral visual fields. Macular or acute vision is used to monitor the specific task at hand as well as to help guide dif-ferent parts of the body that are engaged in the activity. Auditory input (via the cochlear division of VIII, and con-trolled in part by cranial nerves V, VII, IX and X plus cervical musculature) registers sounds resulting from the activity as well as aiding in auditory spatial orientation. Graviceptors throughout the body and the specialized receptors (maculae of the utricle and succulus) of the inner ears continually relay subtle messages concerned with gravity, acceleration, decel-eration and postural adaptations. A multitude of cutaneous, subcutaneous and deeper lying receptors (proprioceptive and visceral) send in signals that relate where each and every part of the body is in relation to itself and to the environment, in-cluding signals that send information concerning velocity of movement, strength, tension, the degree of being «on target» and on and on. Suffice it to say that in any activity performed by the human organism, at least ten pairs of cranial nerves and thirty-one pairs of spinal nerves (and especially those at cervical cord levels), are sending coded messages into the CNS, to a greater or lesser degree, to inform it about the activity in which it is engaged at the moment. It is through this multiple avenue of input, and integrated responses coupled with immediate feedback, that the nervous system «learns» how to perfect skilled patterns of movement (BOWER [12], VOLKMAR & GREENOUGH [52]). The majority of these skills become «semiautomatic» or learned responses and are primarily monitored, integrated and controlled by the «unconscious» levels of the neuraxis.

Once a skill is perfected the conscious brain need not be aware of the vast array of incoming signals, including re-afferent stimuli that are involved in carrying out an activity. It is theorized that most of the «learning» that occurs in the CNS is stored as «patterned engrams» at various hierarchical and overlapping or redundant levels of the neuraxis (GRANIT [23]). An example of this is illustrated in Fig. 19 in relation to the visual system. Over eight hierarchical levels are involved with the storage and control of visual information. These same areas, and others not shown, are also involved with visual-manual, visual-auditory, visual-vestibular, and many other visually coordinated patterns of information storage. These areas not only overlap in reception, storage and retrieval of visual information but they function in cancelling out (inhibiting) or reinforcing (exciting) one another according to the demands placed upon the organism at any given moment. Numerous hierarchical maps could be illustrated to show the overlapping distribution of various nuclei of the neuraxis concerned with auditory input and associative memory, spatiotemporal orientation, somesthetic senses or comprehension and expression of verbal and non-verbal communication, etc.

Can these hierarchical and somewhat redundant polysensory nuclear centers of the CNS give us some insight concerning neuroplasticity and recovery of function following brain injury? I believe that the answer is yes. If we look at these centers and ask «*Why* do they exist?», we may be able to gain

Figure 19. Hierarchical levels involved with the storage and control of visual information.

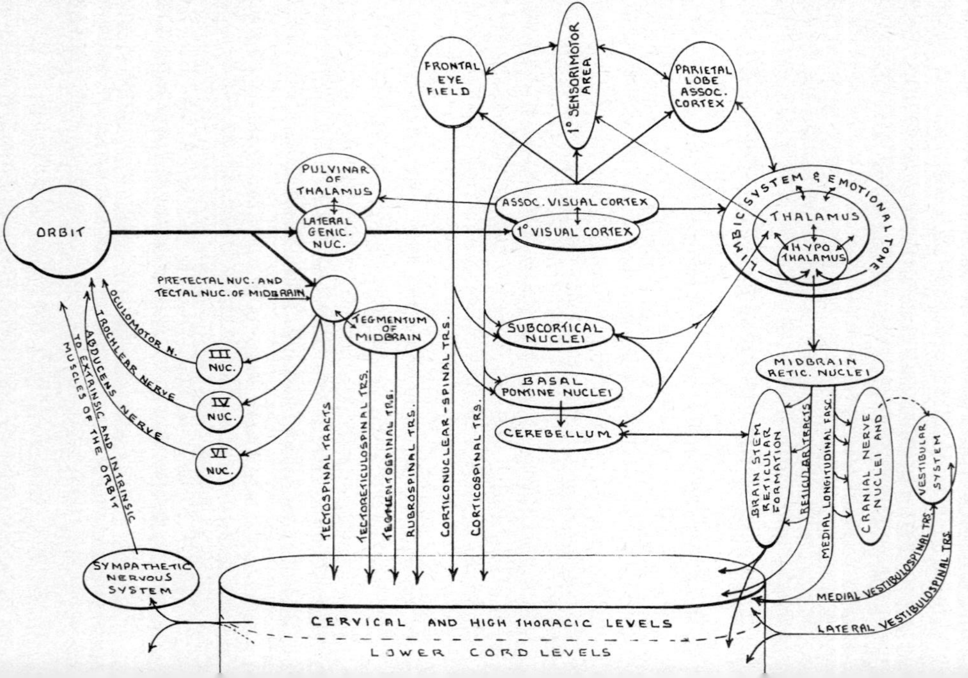

56

some understanding concerning their importance in (re)habilitation. Obviously, these centers are critical to the functional integrity of the organism, and therefore are essential for survival. In thinking about the structure and function in terms of survival, what senses would be necessary for interacting with, «learning» from and surviving in a changing environment? (This assumes that the organism is already endowed with an autonomic nervous system that functions in digestion, respiration, fluid balance, cardiovascular regulation, etc.) The following senses appear to be vital. (1) The organism must have distant and contact receptors, and (2) it must have spatiotemporal orientation both in respect to itself and the environment (HELD [26]). In higher vertebrates, the auditory, visual and flutter-vibratory senses endow animals with distant receptors, while contact or exteroception is provided by numerous types of receptors of which the touch-tactile senses are probably the most important. The spatiotemporal sensors include those already noted above, plus the vestibular and graviceptors of the labyrinths, and graviceptors and general proprioceptors of the rest of the body. These critical senses (of which there appear to be five) are represented by the «star» analogy in Fig. 20. These senses need to have a means whereby they can channel their different inputs into a common polysensory neuron, or pool of neurons, for comparison and integration prior to sending out signals, either to other hierarchical centers, or to lower motoneurons for appropriate responses. These polysensory cells must have some form of memory storage so that the organism can react reflexively with stereotyped patterns of behavior and/or «learn» from experiences through interacting with the environment and responding with less stereotyped behaviors. In order to understand this analogy on a very basic level, one needs to look at primitive creatures, living in the primeval seas. Organisms were able to survive over eons of time with only three primitive senses, vibratory (flutter and vibration), touch and pressure. These senses provided these creatures with distant and contact receptors and spatiotemporal orientation (SARNAT & NETSKY [45]). The distant and contact receptors consisted of ciliated structures or hair cells associated

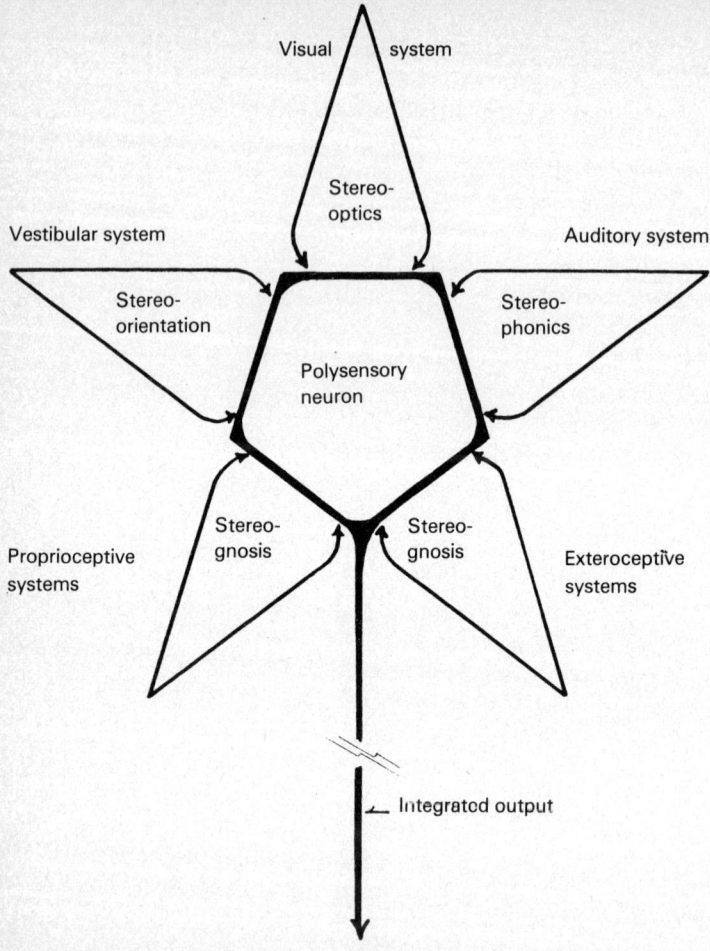

Figure 20. The «star analogy» representing the five critical senses involved in spatiotemporal orientation. Bilateral input is channeled into a polysensory neuron for comparison and integration.

with either a gelatinous-like material or a thin vibrating membrane. These structures are known to be highly sensitive to distant and nearby flutter and vibratory stimuli or pressure waves, depth changes, and touch, and provide the organism with a degree of spatiotemporal orientation. Other types of

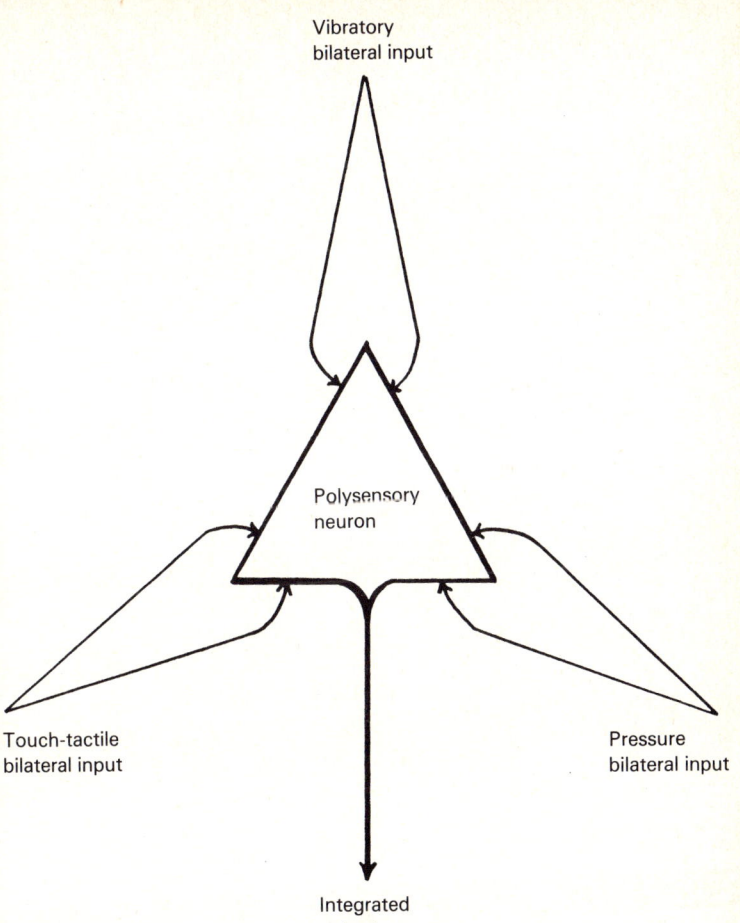

Figure 21. The three primary senses of primitive organisms and a primordial polysensory neuron. This system endowed these creatures with spatiotemporal orientation.

primitive pressure and vibratory sensors, located in and around muscles, fasciae, bones, cartilage or air sacs, and viscera, also endowed these organisms with a sense of spatio-temporal orientation. These senses, sometimes referred to as «vibratory-touch-pressure» receptors, fulfill the criteria that organisms must have spatiotemporal orientation coupled with distant and contact receptors. Later in evolution, a primitive form of hearing and vision developed. Essentially these are highly refined modifications of vibratory receptors or frequency wave detectors.

If we confine our thinking to primitive organisms possessing only vibratory-touch-pressure sensors, then these creatures should have a common ganglionic center or cell type capable of receiving input from these receptor organs for comparing this data, before making a response. This cell would be the primordia of polysensory neurons found in man's CNS (Fig. 21). Throughout evolution as greater differentiation of receptors occurs along with increasing cephalization, segmentation, and variations in responses, the basic need would remain for locating polysensory neurons at various hierarchical centers of the neuraxis for comparison of incoming data that is critical for survival. Chart B illustrates these major nuclear areas of the CNS that appear to have cell populations characteristic of polysensory neurons, i.e., cells that receive multiple «bits» of sensory data from different levels of the neuraxis and are primarily concerned with spatiotemporal orientation, distant and contact information. All of these centers, either via direct or indirect fiber connections are believed to receive, integrate and have «engrams» for storage of visual, auditory, exteroceptive (touch-tactile) data, and proprioceptive (general and special) information. For example, in various association centers of the cerebral cortex information from these senses may be stored in polysensory neurons that are principally concerned with emotional thought processes or «internal» visualization of an event. In primary cortical centers, these five bits of data may be stored as engram patterns principally concerned with visual input (or auditory or somesthetic, etc.). In subcortical nuclei this data might be stored as part of a complex of stereotyped reflexes or as semiautomatic learned responses. At lower brainstem levels they may be stored as engrams associated with visceral or equilibrium responses. Or at cervical levels, they could be stored as reflex/responses associated with spatial orientation (head-on-body patterns) or with contact

Chart B. Major nuclear centers of the CNS that appear to have cell populations characteristic of polysensory neurons.

	Visual system	Auditory system	Exteroceptive touch-tactile system	Proprioceptive system	Vestibular system
Telencephalic cortical levels:					
1° sensorimotor area (4, 3, 1+2)	●		●	●	●
Visual cortex (areas 17, 18, 19)	●	●	●	●	●
Med. temp. lobe parahippocampal area	●	●			?
Lat. temp. lobe auditory assoc area (22+21)	●	●	?	?	●
Superior parietal lobe (areas 5+7)	●		●	●	●
Diencephalic thalamic levels					
Ventral nuclear area (nuc. vent. lat.)			●	●	●
Lateral geniculate nucleus	●	?	?	?	?
Medial geniculate nucleus		●	?	?	?
Pulvinar and lateral nuclear area	●	●	●	●	●
Midbrain superior colliculi (tectum)	●	●	●	●	●
Cerebellar vermis and flocculonodular lobes	●	●	●	●	●
Brain stem trigeminal nuclear system	●	●	●	●	●
Brain stem reticular system	●	●	●	●	●
Spinal cord nucleus proprius			●	●	●

reception such as touch. *Therefore, at various hierarchical levels these five bits of information appear to be stored as engrams in polysensory neurons, not as duplicate patterns, but in relation to the primary function of the center in which they are stored.* For this author, this hypothesis helps explain some of the reasons why the nervous system appears to have overlapping or somewhat redundant functional systems in a hierarchical sense. Also, this adds a needed dimension to the concept of neuroplasticity. In looking at and understanding the nervous system from this perspective one can appreciate the need for and the nature of polysensory neurons within various nuclear centers of the CNS. Continual matching of data from multipotential and multisensory inputs from the total organism must be received and integrated in these nuclear areas. Information that is pertinent at the moment is passed on to higher levels and matched against previously stored memory «engrams», while that which is familiar or well known, is dampened, inhibited or integrated at lower levels.

BACH-y-RITA (1972) has shown that vibratory or tactile stimulation coupled with proprioception can be used as a substitute for vision or hearing. Tactile-proprioceptive senses have been used for decades as a substitute for reading. Blind persons use the tapping of the long, white cane as a radar («sixth») sense for spatial orientation. And HELEN KELLER, once she was taught how to use her remaining senses (vibratory, touch-tactile and proprioceptive systems), could «hear», «see», communicate and interact exceptionally well in her environment in spite of her handicap. These examples, and many more that could be cited, gives one additional insight into the compensatory action of the nervous system, – i.e., receptors can be used in a multipotential manner. Likewise, polysensory neurons and various nuclear centers of the neuraxis including their interconnecting fiber systems and synaptic connections, are endowed to a greater or lesser degree with «alternative potentials». The «star analogy» is used to explain this compensatory or «alternative potential» of the nervous system. If one input source of the star is lost, the four remaining senses can be used for channeling information into polysensory neurons at various levels of the neuraxis. This information will be integrated, though it is only based upon four sources of data, before it is passed on to other centers and re-matched with input that is coming into those centers. Repeated purposeful use of this circuitry over a period of time, along with the possibility that the synaptic sites left vacant by the loss of one input channel will be taken over by one or more of the four remaining inputs and/or cross-over (commissural) fibers (STEIN [48], HELD & FREED-MAN [27], RAISMAN [40]), eventually may help reestablish some balance and functional integrity of these polysensory neurons at various levels of the neuraxis.

In looking in greater depth at the concept of «alternative potentials» one must keep in mind the fact that man is not consciously aware of the vast amount of input continually being received by his total body, yet this information is vital for normal functioning. During growth and development the vast majority of activities engaged in by the infant and child are performed as subcortical (unconscious) reflex/responses, trial and error learning, or by imitation-like responses (RAISMAN [39], RAISMAN & FIELD [41], PAINE, BRAZELTON, DONOVAN, DRORBAUGH, HUBBELL & SEARS [36], BENNETT, DIAMOND, KRECH & ROSENZWEIG [36], GREENOUGH [24], RAISMAN [40]). Similarly, as soon as any conscious purposeful movement pattern is mastered, such as standing, walking, running, or even writing, this activity is quickly «relegated» to unconscious levels and becomes a part of a repertoire of semi-automatic learned responses. By the time the nervous system matures, it has stored within it a vast compilation of subcortical patterned responses, the great majority of which are «unknown» to the conscious nervous system. On the surface this appears to be somewhat of a paradox, i.e., the organism expends a great deal of energy perfecting everything it does, yet in the final analysis it is almost entirely unaware of the multitude of inputs and responses continually occurring within its own nervous system so that it can continue to function normally. For example, in the simple act of holding a pen and writing, the conscious brain is no longer aware of all of the input coming from the digits of the hand holding the pen, or the «contact» and proprioceptive inputs between and among the digits that are adjacent to one another, or the ulnar surface of the hand (and perhaps the forearm) moving across the writing surface, or the fine movements of the digits automatically guiding the formation of each letter being written. Nor is the writer conscious of the total body position involved, or the alignment of the neck that is automatically positioned by the eyes, or the constant scanning and saccadic movements of the visual system automatically checking that which is being written. And though the contralateral hand is not engaged in the writing, it is involved in some activity either by holding the paper, supporting the upper-trunk or perhaps the head, or to some extent, mirror-imaging the hand that is doing the writing. It is interesting to note that if one switches hands and attempts to write with the non-dominate hand, the dominate hand will invariably assume a mirror-image position. Similarly, the way in which the writing paper is positioned (i.e., parallel with the long axis of the forearm-hand that is doing the writing, centered in front of the person, or parallel with the long axis of the forearm-hand that previously did the writing) will determine, in part, whether the person writes normally with the hand and pen lying below or inferior to the words being written, or with the hand hooked or hyperflexed at the wrist and positioned above or superior to the words being written. More importantly, the visual system automatically positions the neck so that the head is cocked at an appropriate angle for monitoring the writing and the writing hand. With this realignment of the cervical axis by the visual system, the trunk is automatically realigned to compensate for the head tilting. This is a simple demonstration of basic patterns of bilaterality of function and the integrative action of the nervous system at subcortical levels. This also shows how the visual-manual systems primarily pre-set or automatically determine the realignment of the entire body in preparation for and during the performance of an activity. One could go on and on and note the position of each joint of the body, the input coming from the gluteal area, the lower limbs, or even the auditory system monitoring the «scratching» noise as the pen moves on the paper. The point here is that the entire body is engaged in the act of writing, even though the conscious brain is not aware of all of the input that is necessary for setting the background postural tone and adjustments that enables one to write. Yet it is this «background» input of bilateral stability-mobility patterns, along with the continual ongoing activity taking place at every level of the neuraxis, that is critical for normal functioning, and becomes especially critical in regard to (re)habilitation.

The nuclear centers monitoring all of the activity involved in writing, or in any activity, are the same ones that were involved in perfecting normal patterns of movement and postural tone when the organism was learning to raise its head, roll over, get up into the all-fours position, rock back and forth, crawl, knee-stand or squat-sit, and eventually cruise and walk. Within these hierarchical nuclear centers, which undoubtedly include the primary receptor-effector centers of the cerebral cortex, are chemical memory circuits, likened to the star analogy, that are concerned with the storage of patterns of movement and posture. As these centers mature along with the entire nervous system, and certain postural adaptations are repeated over and over again, some circuits and synaptic connections apparently become «dominant» while other circuits appear to be relegated to a «recessive» role or are over-ridden by higher centers and in turn are controlled in part by newer pathways (GRANIT [23]). In other words, as higher level functions develop along with myelination of newer pathways, dendritic growth, and maturation of synaptic knobs, the older pathways that once performed a patterned response are no longer vital for carrying out a particular activity pattern. This is not to say that these older routes die out or fade away. They remain, and function in the normal individual in maintaining the overall integrity of the nervous system. However they function in a minor way in comparison to the newer pathways that carry out most of the highly refined purposeful learned activities in which man engages. When higher functions are lost or damaged due to brain injury, the older, once utilized recessive or alternate routes remain. If these can be «tapped» or strengthened, by using them in the same way, or in a manner similar to the way that they were originally used, then these older pathways may constitute viable «alternative potentials» through which functional improvements may be gained. (Remember that the phylogenetic and ontogenetically older or archi pathways of the lower brain stem, spinal cord and archicerebellum were once the major circuits for «controlling» our midline or axial postural stability-mobility patterns.) As the intermediate or paleo-systems of the upper brain stem-paleocerebellar circuits developed, they dampened down or inhibited the older centers, and at the same time added a finer degree of control over the axial body along with control of the proximal limb structures. With maturity of the telencephalic-diencephalic nuclear areas and neocerebellar centers, control was gained over all of the afore-mentioned areas (principally by inhibition or cortical over-ride), along with fine control of the distal limb structures. Along with this, another dimension was added to the control of the body, i.e., speed, dexterity and individualized patterns of behavior via the «pyramidal system».) In brain injury these «added refinements» endowed by the neo-cortical systems are usually the most severely involved. The inhibitory overlay which they provided over the older systems, and upon which the older systems have become dependent for their functional integrity, is disrupted or lost. When the lower centers are released from interaction with higher centers they are no longer capable of functioning as they once did during growth and development, i.e., they gradually lose their full potential for controlling functional patterns of movement due to their long term reliance upon higher level inputs for their control. In other words, they have become minor or non-dominant systems in regard to controlling patterns of purposeful behavior. (The younger the organism is at the time of brain injury, the greater is the chance that the older systems are still dominant or less differentiated and therefore can aid in recovery of function. Case in point, the right hemisphere (Area 45–44 or Broca's convolution) taking over motor speech functions, or a contralateral WERNICKE's area taking over receptive speech functions following a lesion to the left hemisphere, or the switching of hand dominance following brain injury.)

The question is, can these older circuits be utilized and strenghtened in order to regain some degree of functional improvement following brain injury? The answer to this depends upon a multitude of variables, some of which are (1) the state of CNS maturity at the time of insult; (2) the extent of the lesion as well as the location (cortical, higher and lower level subcortical nuclear centers and fiber pathways, internal capsule, brain stem, etc.) (3) time lapsed between the time of the insult and the beginning of rehabilitation and therefore the amount of sensory deprivation and/or mal-adaptive processes that have occurred; (4) whether or not the «memory circuits» of the limbic system are damaged; (5) the individual's pre-morbid personality, talents, drives, etc., (6) the health of the individual; and (7) the cause of the brain injury, i.e., traumatic or mechanical, vascular, metastatic, toxic or infectious, etc. However, assuming that we are not concerned here with patients that are decerebrate (vegetative), but with those that have a potential for returning to society, then I believe that the answer to this basic question is «yes», i.e., the older circuitry can be «tapped» and gradually strengthened so that it can be utilized as a means of regaining functional improvement. However, these older CNS systems cannot be «re-awakened» by utilizing techniques that are applicable for rehabilitating the neo-systems, i.e., the use of therapeutic measures that require a degree of conscious effort such as walking, dressing, writing, eating, speaking, etc. Rather, these older systems need to be tapped and reinforced by having the patient use them in the manner in which they once functioned, i.e., as subcortical or unconscious *bilateral* primitive patterns of stability with limited mobility. Along with this, external reinforcement must be given to the patient. This is done by utilizing the more primitive kinds of stimuli, such as vibration, touch, pressure and resistance, coupled with enough external control so that feedback from the movement patterns are as nearly normal as possible. All of this stimuli is given at an increased level of intensity in order to help «re-awaken» and reinforce the circuitry that is being utilized. With repeated use of these kinds of techniques over a period of time, the older centers, fiber tracts and synapses, at various levels of the neuraxis, appear to regain a degree of bilateral control over the basic functional patterns, including those concerned with balance, coordination, synergy, and timing of movement. Once these are integrated and «ingrained» into the CNS, less primitive bilateral patterns of movement can be used in the (re)habilitative process along with external stimuli that will help to reinforce the learning process at this functional level. This technique of (re)habilitation parallels our own growth and development, including all of the external reinforcements or «hard knocks» that each of us endured from various kinds of stimuli, as we matured, and which helped us perfect our own coordinated patterns of behavior.

In summary, the NS receives multisensory input from multipotential receptors located in every part of the body. During any activity in which the body engages, at least 30 pairs of spinal nerves and a minimum of 10 cranial nerves are transmitting coded messages from their various receptors into a variety of hierarchical polysensory nuclear areas of the CNS. These centers continually compare these afferent and re-afferent messages with data that has been stored from the past, i.e., genetico-environmental influences. The momentary circumstances of the present and the immediate future is also compared. These multiple bits of coded input are matched and re-integrated, then re-coded, and transmitted to adjacent centers and/or to craniospinal motoneurons for appropriate responses, which includes the vital re-afferent input in relation to the response. With repeated use of various stability-mobility patterns, over a prolonged period of time, various nuclear centers and their respective pathways are believed to become dominant. Speed and agility of movement is perfected along with a tendency toward lateralization of function, especially in regard to handedness, and the speech center of the brain (perhaps some forms of auditory and visual acuity), and some aspects of the emotional components of behavior. In spite of this trend, the organism primarily functions throughout life as a bilaterally organized or stereomorphophysiological system. By recognizing this avenue of approach to rehabilitation, i.e., initiating therapy at the lower levels of function in relation to the bilateral multisensory and polysensory systems before ever attempting to rehabilitate the higher more lateralized and specialized levels of function, I believe that therapy has made some of its most important gains.

In actuality, the plasticity of the nervous system has always been known to the nervous system! However, it remains for man to discover ways to optimally utilize these plastic potentials. Now that science has «discovered» CNS plasticity and is gaining a better understanding of the maturation and functional potentials of hierarchical and polysensory systems, coupled with awareness of the effects of sensory deprivation on the CNS, the future or rehabilitation is more promising than ever before.

The ten cardinal principles of (re)habilitation

1. Prevention of sensory deprivation
2. Active participation
3. Repetition with and without variation
4. Meaningful
5. Motivation
6. «Forcing»
7. Cervicocephalocaudal law of development
8. Subcortical integration precedes cortical integration
9. Facilitation/inhibition
10. Patience and T.L.C.

I consider these to be cardinal principles, based in part upon years of experience by clinicians and upon common sense. Many of these have been used for ages by man and other animals in teaching and/or for self-learning. They are also based upon research that has shown that these parameters are vital for normal nervous system integration, maturation and survival of the organism in the environment. The research literature supporting these principles will not be noted in depth as it is not the intention of the author to write an extensive review on each of these subjects. A «Bibliography of Related Readings» will be found at the end of this section for those who desire additional information. These principles are not listed in order of importance. All of them play an important role in normal (mental and physical) growth, development and learning as well as in (re)habilitation. Each principle will be discussed briefly in order to explain its role in relation to recovery of function following brain injury.

1. Prevention of sensory deprivation

The research literature of the past three decades has presented a vast amount of data concerning the short and long term effects of sensory deprivation (S.D.). S.D. is defined here in its broadest sense, i.e., any change in the internal or external environment that deprives an organism of normal and necessary sensorimotor, re-afferent stimuli. (See also Chapter 4 by ROSENZWEIG.) This includes the isolation normally found in the «sterile environment» of an intensive care unit, private room or hospital; the lack of familiar surroundings; separation from loved ones and visitors coupled with loss of familiar sounds such as music, traffic or street noises and vibrations, etc.; the excessive use of prescribed drugs for sedation and/or medication combined with interruptions of REM sleep, especially at night; confinement to a bed (or isolette); a change in food, fluid and even the air that one breathes; and last but not least, lack of movement and therefore loss or diminution of normal feedback from the exteroproprioceptive systems of the body, especially those involved in spatiotemporal orientation. The effects of S.D. on the nervous system has been likened to that of muscles deprived of normal functions, i.e., the gradual loss of muscle tone and eventual atrophy of muscle fibers following prolonged disuse. In the sensorially deprived nervous system, one sees a similar diminution of function in the neo-systems, especially those that are concerned with recent memory and cognition. Also there are usually decided changes in emotional tone. Undoubtedly, this is a reflection of the changes that occur in the reticulolimbic system, a functional part of the CNS that is extremely vulnerable to anesthetics, tranquilizers, pain medications, changes in normal sleep patterns, awake and altering patterns and loss of stimuli that are necessary for keeping the organism functioning as normally as possible. The reticulolimbic system is believed to be responsible for our emotional tone (behavioral patterns), drives or motivations, short and long term memory storage and retrieval of knowledge or cognition. In other words, it is a vital regulator of the CNS that is necessary for homeostasis as well as for maintaining the functional integrity of the entire nervous system. Like the triceps brachii and the quadraceps muscles that are usually the most susceptible to change resulting from disuse, the reticulolimbic system undergoes comparable anatomical and physiological changes due to S.D. These alterations are believed to occur initially at the area of the synapses. Any lesion of the nervous system upsets the functional integrity of the system. When this is compounded with S.D., it is theorized that the prognosis for recovery of function is poorer than when precautions are taken to prevent S.D. Granted, there are limitations as to what one can do to prevent S.D. especially with severely injured patients or those who have had rather massive CVA's. However, even with severely involved patients, be they comatose, semicomatose, or semiconscious, the reticulolimbic system, along with the muscular system can be stimulated in such a way that excessive S.D. can be prevented. For example, if this author were asked to design an ICU for these kinds of patients, the following equipment and therapeutic measures would be useful: (1) The patient's bed would be equipped with a vibrator that is capable of vibrating the mattress. A small computer would activate the vibrator at varying intervals and also at different frequencies (100–350 Hz range). For brief moments the frequency would drop below 50 Hz, preferably into the 1 to 26 Hz range in order to cause an alerting reaction in the reticular system. (2) The bed would be mechanized so that it would gradually flex and extend the knees, hips, trunk, and neck, and if possible gently shift the person slightly from one side to another. (3) Music interspersed with everyday noises of traffic, conversations and recordings of the voices of loved ones and friends would be piped into the room at odd intervals during the day. This would be varied so that loud sharp alerting sounds as well as soft or far away noises (dogs barking in the distance or the passing of an airplane overhead) would be an integral part of the music and voices. (4) At least two or more times a day a trained therapist would stimulate the major functional muscle groups by moving the limbs passively through the range of motion and by using a vibrator (100–350 Hz range) for activating the tonic vibratory reflexes (TVR) of the various muscle groups of the body. During this time the therapist would talk to the patient, varying her tone and changing the pitch of her voice. (5) All personnel entering the room would be instructed to talk to the patient and repeatedly touch them or hold their hand, arm, or shoulder, always using firm, but gentle, pressure. (6) The temperature and lighting conditions in the room would be varied to stimulate a more normal environment, and occasionally various odors would be used to help activate the patient's reticulolimbic system. Once the individual is out of ICU, appropriate therapeutic techniques would be instituted immediately. In the meantime, these measures should help prevent the long and short term effects of sensory deprivation and help maintain the functional integrity of the nervous system. In effect, these techniques are stimulating the basic needs of the patient's nervous system, i.e., the older or more primitive senses of feedback from movement, the vibratory-touch-pressure receptors, as well as the special senses of smell, sound and vestibular input.

2. Active participation

The nervous system learns by doing. Active involvement has repeatedly been shown to be superior to passive participation in order for the nervous system to learn, mature and remain viable. Granted, one can learn by observation but this has never been as effective as learning actively. The organism needs to «get into the act» so to speak, and go through the process of an activity before permanent memory engrams are laid down. Also, learning occurs faster when multiple senses are used, instead of just one or two. In other words, when total body movements are involved in the learning process along with visual and auditory input and perhaps odor from the surrounding environment, optimal learning occurs. In rehabilitation it is necessary at times to use passive treatment techniques in order to prevent contractures, atrophy and general deterioration. However, every effort should be made to get the patient actively involved in the (re)habilitation process so that the patient learns how to carry out purposeful and sequential movement patterns. This is one of the advantages in using therapeutic techniques based upon developmental sequences. The total body is always involved bilaterally, symmetrically and reciprocally, along with midline stability-mobility patterns. Interestingly, these techniques are some of the best ways known for a person to begin to «know» their body. Most individuals are not aware of their own body in relation to feedback from forces and patterns of movement, the effects of gravity, posture and balance mechanisms, or their individualistic use of the visual and auditory systems, or even of foot dominance patterns. This is not surprising in light of how the nervous system develops and functions. Probably 99% of everything we do, see, hear, feel, smell, etc. is integrated automatically at subcortical levels. This enables us to function optimally when we are normal, but it can be devastating following a nervous system lesion, especially when movement patterns, sensory perceptions and/or spatiotemporal orientation are disrupted. However, therapeutic techniques that enable the patient to utilize total developmental body patterns (such as mat exercises or rolling over, the all-fours position for rocking back and forth diagonally, crawling, etc., the Bobath ball, Ayers scooter board, and similar techniques) enables the nervous system to begin to reorganize itself subcortically as it is forced to respond to more normalized bilateral patterns of movement. Comparably, perceiving multisensory input from extensive parts of the body is preferable to just one or a few senses.

The best way in which a person can begin to appreciate therapeutic techniques based upon developmental sequence and/or normal reflex/responses, is to perform them, preferably with vision occluded. This forces the normal individual to appreciate a multitude of bodily senses and especially the feedback or re-afferent input that lets one know where each part of the body is in relation to all other parts. One begins to perceive the forces that are impinging upon different body surfaces including one's joints, and a perspective of the body in relation to the total spatiotemporal environment. This active participation also helps one appreciate why different therapeutic techniques are used in (re)habilitation and what these techniques are attempting to do for the nervous system of the brain-injured patient.

3. Repetition with and without variation

Obviously, in order to learn a skill or memorize something, one must repeat the process over and over until it becomes a permanent part of one's abilities. The same is true in (re)habilitation of patients with some exceptions. In many cases the patient lacks the drive, energy and/or the ability to repeat a process a sufficient number of times in order to improve performance. Also, recovery following brain injury can be a long, slow and tedious process, somewhat resembling our formative years during our own growth, development and maturation. The patient can become discouraged or bored rather readily in comparison to a normal individual. Coupled with this is the fact that the nervous system adapts[1] and habituates[2] to that which is too repetitive or consistent. It begins to ignore or inhibit stimuli, especially when it is constant, aberrant or meaningless. It is believed that the reticulolimbic system is primarily involved in this process, just as it is involved in the activating and alerting mechanisms that keep an organism viable. Fortunately, the reticulolimbic system is one of the easiest to «activate» or reach with various therapeutic treatment techniques. This is because of its archi or primitive nature, i.e., it has multiple efferent and afferent connections with all other systems of the CNS. It readily reacts to change and in so doing restimulates other nuclear centers, by changing cell thresholds, so that these areas can react more appropriately to stimuli. In any therapeutic techniques that utilizes repetitive patterns of stimuli and/or movement patterns, there should be a sufficient variation or change incorporated into the technique to prevent the CNS from adapting or habituating and thus depriving it from gaining some improvement from the therapeutic process. Variation can be something that is as simple as giving the patient a

[1] *Adaptation* in the nervous system is seen when a sense organ adjusts to the intensity of, or quality of, a stimulation.

[2] Habituation is concerned with the organisms ability to become accustomed to a stimulus, i.e., having the ability to effect a tolerance to a quantity or quality of stimuli because of habitual or continued use.

quick command with the voice suddenly raised, to more subtle forms of changing the person's perception of verticality, putting them slightly off balance, tapping or vibrating the group of muscles being resisted, or any number of techniques that alerts the system. No matter what is used, it is the therapist who must remain alert and change the stimulus parameters in order to prevent the patient's nervous system from habituating to the techniques being used.

It should be noted that there are many occasions when habituation and adaptation can be a beneficial part of the (re)habilitation process. This is especially true for patients that have hypertonicity and/or are hyperkinetic, tense or irritable. Repetitive patterns, such as gentle rocking, slow rolling and slow rhythmical soft sounds or stroking patterns, are not only soothing to the nervous system, but they tend to relax and inhibit emotional and muscular tone. When judiciously used, these techniques can put a patient to sleep, as they once did for many of us when we were infants and were held and gently rocked back and forth.

4. Meaningful

In order for learning to occur in the nervous system, that which is learned must have some meaning or degree of importance to the organism that is doing the learning. If the system cannot perceive certain forms of stimuli or cannot relate to them in some purposeful way, it can either ignore the stimuli, or prevent memory storage from occurring, unless perhaps, trauma is involved. This phenomenon of the nervous system has been experienced by all of us. It has been repeatedly demonstrated with animals that are exposed, for the first time, to a mirror. Initially, the animal will attempt to interact with the image in the mirror. However, in a relatively short time it will give up and ignore it or overtly avoid its presence. Only once did I observe an animal (feline domesticus) repeatedly use a mirror or the reflection from a window or glass door to an advantage. This was an albino cat that I adopted into my household. He was deaf, had poor vision and was extremely fearful of his environment, which included several other cats, a dog and a raccoon, all of which got along well except on occasions when they would torment one another. Somehow this cat learned that if he sat facing a large mirror or glass door he could observe the entire surroundings behind him including parts of adjacent rooms. In this way he kept track of the whereabouts of everyone. No longer could another animal stealthily creep up on him and surprise him. Once he learned this he acclimated to the household and lost many of his fears, including being the lowest member of the pecking order. This animal utilized these reflections because they had significance directly related to his survival instincts. Similarly, in therapy, as in life, the more closely the event or learning situation parallels or is related in some way to survival mechanisms the better one learns. (The term «survival mechanisms» is used here in its broadest connotation, i.e., basic survival instincts, genetically endowed reflex/responses and patterns of movement, as well as psychosocial drives, such as to achieve, to be acceptable to somebody or to love and be loved.) In any therapeutic exercise or treatment technique the patient needs to understand why something is being done or why she or he is engaged in a certain activity. Also, activities utilized in therapy must be meaningful to the patient's nervous system, i.e., it needs to be based upon normal physiological reflex/responses or sequential sensorimotor movement patterns. For example, it is of little value to have a patient flex and extend or rotate an isolated part of an extremity over and over in an attempt to regain function, because the nervous system is not organized in this manner. It functions and learns in relation to total bilateral and reciprocal patterns of movement and usually in response to some meaningful stimulus complex. Therefore all activities in which the patient engages or is engaged in should have some relationship to the needs of the nervous system and to the realistic goals of the patient and/or those who may have to care for the individual.

5. Motivation

The reticulolimbic system is believed to be the major center of the CNS that controls and regulates man's emotional tone, his abilities to lay down memories and retrieve them, and his drives. Trauma of any kind can readily upset this system, depressing the emotional tone as well as the forces that drive us to eat, sleep, work, play, achieve and be gregarious individuals. Any loss of self-motivation of and by itself can be traumatic to an individual. When it is coupled with a brain lesion, an inability to move normally and/or perceive certain kinds of stimuli, it can be devastating. One of the major goals in (re)habilitation is to motivate the patient over a long enough period of time until self-motivation is restored. This process of external motivation must be reality oriented and not based upon false hopes and promises. Also, it needs to be a step-by-step procedure, i.e., setting short-term goals so that the patient can achieve them in a relatively brief period of time. An example of this might be learning to roll over, or sit up, or move the extremities through the range of motion in a smooth sequential manner or just re-gaining strength. Along with this the clinician and/or therapist must project a genuine feeling of care for the patient, including an ability to motivate the patient. At the same time the clinician needs to recognize when the patient begins to reestablish self-esteem and a renewed drive to succeed. It is at this time that the therapist must be prepared to step aside and terminate the dependency the patient has on him/her and reinforce the patient's positive drives. The major exception to this is when the patient is motivated to remain dependent upon the clinician or therapist and/or stay in the secure environment of the hospital or rehabilitation facility. This situation can be handled by trained personnel or by the individuals who have worked closely with the patient. The goal is to continually recognize and reinforce the patient's healthy drives and inhibit the negative nonreality oriented behavioral patterns. Another factor concerning motivation of the patient needs to be mentioned. This deals with those members of the family and/or friends of the patient who are reality oriented. These individuals need to be included, as much as is possible, in the (re)habilitation process in order to assist them in understanding and accepting the patient, helping the patient become positively motivated and in planning realistic long-term goals.

6. Forcing

The concept of «forcing» is not a new one. It has been used in (re)habilitation for many years but with different definitions and connotations. For example, the use of resistance or adding weights to the limbs has been used for ages in strengthening muscles, increasing range of motion, or decreasing abnormal movement patterns. These could all be considered techniques of «forcing the system» to work harder or more appropriately. Another type of forcing has been used in psychological rehabilitation of patients, i.e., setting standards that must be achieved or adhered to. The term is used here, however, in a slightly different manner and is related to an inherent property of nervous system functioning. As previously stated, the nervous system utilizes multipotential and multisensory stimuli in order to function normally. As long as all of the senses are functioning the system will depend upon these for its needs. Even when one (or more) senses are changed, due to CNS insult or the aging process, it will usually continue to rely upon these senses even though they are no longer functioning normally. It is only when a sense is completely lost that the system will, in some way, enhance the functional abilities of the remaining senses and begin to substitute them for that which is lost. A case in point is the following that should be actively performed by everyone who works in a rehabilitation center. Wear a blindfold, that occludes all vision and light, for a period of time, preferably 24 hours, along with one rule that must be followed ... no verbal communication is allowed on the part of the blindfolded person. (This forces the experimentor to rely upon his auditory system for spatiotemporal orientation and not for language communication.) Initially, whether the experimenter is aware of it or not, he will try to keep his eyes open under the blindfold in an attempt to «see». Once he decides that this is foolish he will keep his eyes closed but will inwardly attempt to visualize his environment. It is not until he completely «gives up» his ability to see (externally and internally) and communicate verbally, that he will begin to rely upon his remaining senses and learn to use them for moving about and exploring his surroundings. This is the concept of «forcing» the nervous system to utilize the other senses optimally. For some individuals it takes about a half hour to an hour to begin to consciously realize the tremendous potentials that are available through the remaining senses for moving about and appreciating the environment with the remaining senses. It is my belief that no normal person can truly appreciate and utilize this concept of forcing until they have experienced this situation, simply because of the way in which our nervous systems function.

As previously stated, most of the stimuli received from our environment never reaches consciousness. Yet we are subcortically dependent upon these subliminal inputs for normal function. But paradoxically, we can never become aware of these subliminal stimuli and what they do for us unless we are forced to appreciate them by depriving ourselves of one or more of our vital senses. The same is true in the (re)habilitation of the nervous system. As long as there remains any functional part of a sensory system or movement pattern, no matter if it is essentially useless or handicapping to the individual, the person will automatically rely upon it even if it is detrimental to the persons' progress and recovery process. Because this is an inherent property of the nervous system, it needs to be recognized by everyone who works in rehabilitation. Another way of emphasizing this point is to recognize that some patients will not accept or follow through on prescribed exercises based upon developmental theories (such as reciprocal crawling, knee standing and balancing, rolling over, prone on elbows, etc.) if they can ambulate, even though this proves to be a slow, awkward, stiff-gaited pattern. Few people will learn to lip read or wear a hearing aid if they can catch a phrase or two from someone shouting at them, or until some other circumstance forces them to do so. The partially sighted will not learn to use their «sixth radar sense» for getting around as long as they still have some remaining vision. Therefore, as long as any potential function remains in a given sensorimotor system, the organism will continue to rely upon it and find a multitude of behavioral mechanisms for covering up or compensating for the disability. Few learn to utilize other more viable sensorimotor systems and substitute these for perceiving and functioning optimally in their environment unless they are forced to do so. The principle of forcing the nervous system to use viable alternative systems should be used in (re)habilitation whenever and wherever it is applicable. Not using it may be one of the reasons for our so-called «failures» in rehabilitation. Often times we are too soft on the nervous system, probably because we are incapable of fully comprehending all of its potentials, and therefore we have failed to make it function optimally by forcing it to rely upon alternative sensorimotor systems. Instead, we have relied upon that which remains even though it may be a poor second in comparison to the gains that could have been made with sensory substitution techniques (GRANIT [23]).

7. Cervicocephalocaudal law of development

Even though this law has been spoken to in an earlier part of this chapter, it is listed here because it is one of the cardinal principles of (re)habilitation. Not enough research has been done in the past to examine the importance of the cervical area of the body and the role it plays in normal perception and function. Fortunately a group at Queen's University (Kingston, Ontario, Canada) is undertaking an intensive investigation of this area in the cat, not only in relation to nervous system pathways, receptors and movement, but also in regard to physiological mechanisms such as spatiotemporal orientation, various anatomical considerations and the histochemistry of the muscles of the neck (ABRAHAMS [1], ABRAHAMS, RICHMOND & ROSE [3, 4], ABRAHAMS, RANCIER & ROSE [2]). Their research is helping to substantiate earlier theories based upon pre and post natal development and reflexology, phylogenetic studies of the nervous system, archi, paleo, and neo ascending and descending pathways in man's nervous system that primarily influence cervical levels, and (re)habilitation techniques that are used for gaining midline (especially cervical) stability-mobility patterns. The importance of this area of the body cannot be minimized. It should be considered as the «key» to the total rehabilitation process in that this area controls the head and in so doing enables the special senses therein located to function optimally. These in turn, along with the neck, control the rest of the body. Though this area should always be considered as the primary «target» of the (re)habilitation process, it is never (re)habilitated of and by itself but always in relation to normalized total body reflex/response patterns.

8. Subcortical integration precedes cortical integration

«Beginner's luck» is a phrase often used when a person attempts a new sport or skill for the first time. Much to the surprise of everyone, including the person, there is success. However, when the individual decides to perfect this newfound skill, his luck vanishes. All of us have experienced this at one time or another and especially the frustration involved when we decide to perfect the new activity. We are reluctant to give up, so we try harder. And the harder we try, or the more cortically involved we become, the poorer are the results. What has happened? Unbeknownest to many of us, who like to drive our nervous system cortically, we forget that the system has an amazing facility (once it matures) to organize itself subcortically. It continually performs highly skilled functions for us, especially when it is released from «cortical overdrive». In fact, «cortical overdrive» can be a powerful inhibitor of skill, in that too much conscious effort usually causes unnecessary tensions resulting in lowered performance. In the brain-injured individual a conscious effort to move a part or perform an activity usually results in increased muscle tone, decreased range of motion and increased abnormal movement patterns. Also cortical or conscious driving of the nervous system proves to be a tedious and exhausting job (Brodal [14]). However, if one relaxes and lets the subconscious or semiautomatic reflex/responses take over, the results are superior and energy is conserved. In other words, the older parts of the nervous system that are responsible for integrated patterns of movement in response to purposeful stimuli will function automatically if allowed to do so. Many of the therapeutic techniques used in rehabilitation are based upon this principle, i.e., subcortical re-integration must precede cortical re-integration. Therefore, instead of giving a command to a patient and telling him to perform a specific task, the patient is positioned, resisted, and/or assisted in moving through a total body integrated movement pattern. This is done in such a way that the desired activity is performed automatically. Oftentimes additional stimuli (such as tapping, vibration, pressure, stretching, and especially resistance) are given to specific muscle groups in order to enhance performance. Cortical commands may be used to direct the attention of the patient away from the specific activity being performed and focus the patient's attention on another aspect of the treatment. Such commands as «look up», «don't let me push you off balance», «watch me», «hold on», «go to the end of the mat and come back», etc. are frequently used in this regard. Every attempt is made to prevent the patient from performing cortically. These techniques closely parallel the way in which all of us learned to crawl, cruise, walk, and eventually perform semiskilled movements like eating, dressing, running, etc. We did not consciously or cortically drive each limb or hand as we attempted to get up in the all-fours position and crawl. No thought was given as to how we managed to get up from a sitting position into standing and then walking. Instead we were goal oriented and reached out, and cruised or toddled toward some person or object that held our attention. With repeated trials and some errors, and always stimulated by different goals, we perfected our new-found skills. Conscious cortical drive, specifically related to the performance of a new skill, did not enter the picture until we had spent a few years integrating and perfecting our basic movement patterns. Once achieved, these semiautomatic learned reflex/responses became the foundation upon which newer and more cortically driven activities were added. By understanding how the nervous system progresses through these developmental and integrative stages, a greater appreciation is gained for those therapeutic techniques that are based upon these premises, i.e., subcortical integration precedes cortical integration.

9. Facilitation/inhibition

Fundamental physiological properties of an isolated neuron are facilitation and inhibition. Once a neuron fires an action potential, it does so in an all or none manner, either facilitating or inhibiting other neurons, glands or muscle fibers. However, in the integrative action of the nervous system there are a multitude of subtle changes occurring in the membrane potentials of the different parts of a given neuron. This is especially so in regard to the neuromuscular system, where one sees a subtle balance or gradation occurring between these two forces, i.e., a decrease of tone in one set of muscles and an enhancement or increased tone in the opposing set. A good analogy is the teeter-totter with facilitation sitting at one end and inhibition at the other (Fig. 22). Depending upon the stimulus complex and the needs of the body at any given moment, the teeter-totter constantly undergoes subtle changes in order to maintain the proper balance between these two opposing forces. Following brain injury this balance is upset. Some muscle groups are hypertonic, others hypotonic, with the antigravity muscles usually being more extensively involved. Treatment techniques used in (re)habilitation, as in some of the experimental neurosurgical and pharmacological approaches, attempt to reestablish this critical facilitory-in-

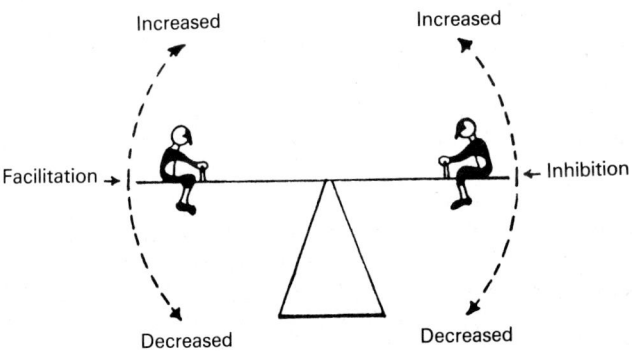

Figure 22. The teeter-totter analogy concerning facilitation and inhibition. (See text for explanation.)

hibitory balance in order to regain muscle synergy. In some techniques the treatment is specifically designed to inhibit one group of muscles while facilitating the opposite group, or shunting the tone into the antagonist. In other techniques, it is to inhibit, as much as possible, an undesirable total body primitive reflex pattern while attempting to facilitate a more normal response. This might be as «simple» a procedure as gaining total body relaxation before attempting movement, or positioning a patient in such a way that the upper limbs automatically extend in response to a sudden external movement that changes the person's center of gravity. At all times a variety of techniques must be used throughout the rehabilitation process in order to continually match, and enhance, the patient's progress. Likewise, the therapist must monitor, and be ready to counteract, any imbalances that may occur between the delicately rebalanced forces of the facilitory/inhibitory teeter-totter. This technique constitutes the art of therapy. The experienced clinician somehow feels, sees or almost intuitively knows the proper stimulus complex to use at any given moment in order to help reestablish, maintain and/or strengthen the gains that have been made. Coupled with this is a «knowing» of just when and how best to force the patient yet another step forward in the (re)habilitation process.

10. Patience and T.L.C.

Adult man is an impatient beast! By the time the brain matures, each person will have established his or her own pace for accomplishing different tasks. To a degree, man can compromise these inherent rhythms and slow down, or speed up, in order to work or keep pace with others. However, in the majority of cases this rhythm tends to dominate us. This can lead to inner frustrations or overt expressions of incompatability. In rehabilitation of the brain-injured we are constantly faced with this problem, as is the patient. The «patience of Job» is needed by all parties concerned because the progress of rehabilitation is usually a long and tedious affair. As the patient grows weary, so does the clinician. This is especially so in cases that take months or years before a small measure of progress is demonstrated. The «light at the end of the tunnel» is in consciously realizing that there are those cases where it may take months to years before the nervous system reestablishes some meaningful synapses and circuitry and begins to regain a more normal balance, – just as it took years for our own systems to mature before our brains were able to function optimally. In other cases, the patient may plateau for an extended period of time and show little to no gains, similar to that which occurs in the normal person during the learning of a new subject or perfecting a new skill. (And there are those cases where no known therapeutic technique can make a substantial improvement in the patient's well being.) However, it is a fact that the nervous system is plastic. It can and does change, though imperceptively, from moment to moment throughout the lifetime of the individual. Extensive scientific data still eludes us concerning how these biochemical and submicroscopic changes occur; nevertheless, they are occurring. Because we cannot readily see or measure them as yet on the crude scales of sciences does not mean that we can deny their existence.

Patience is necessary, along with a certain amount of faith, in knowing that with the proper treatment techniques we are causing changes in the patient's nervous system during and following each therapy session. These facilitation/inhibition techniques (or whatever name they are called by) are attempting to prevent sensory deprivation. At the same time they are forcing the system to actively undergo meaningful reorganization, primarily at subcortical levels. By adding the correct amount of T.L.C. (Tender-Loving-Care) the patient may become self-motivated to the extent that he/she will continue to carry out various prescribed treatments and gradually improve, or at least maintain, the progress that was gained while undergoing active therapy.

Bibliography of readings related to the ten cardinal principles of rehabilitation

AGRAWAL, H.C., FOX, M.W., HIMWICH, W.A.: Neurochemical and behavioral effects of isolation-rearing in the dog. The Sciences (London) *6*, 71–78, 1967.

APPEL, S.H., DAVIS, W., SCOTT, S.: Brain Polysomes: Response to environmental stimulation. Sci. *157,* 836–838, 1967.

BALL, W., TRONICK, E.: Infant responses to impending collison: optical and real. Sci. *171,* 818–820, 1971.

BLAKEMORE, C., COOPER, G.R.: Development of the brain depends on the visual environment. Nature *228,* 477–478, 1970.

BONDY, S.C., DAVID, F.N.: Reversible responses of the cerebral circulation to visual deprivation. Br.Res. *43,* 606–609, 1972.

BONDY, S.C., MORELOS, B.S.: Stimulus deprivation and cerebral blood flow. Exper.Neurol. *31,* 200–206, 1971.

CRAGG, B.G.: The effects of vision and dark-rearing on the size and density of synapses in the lateral geniculate nucleus measured by electron microscopy. Br.Res. *13,* 53–67, 1969.

FIFKOVA, E.: Changes in the visual cortex of rats after unilateral deprivation. Nature *220,* 379–381, 1968.

FREEDMAN, D.G.: Constitutional and environmental interactions in rearing of four breeds of dogs. Sci. *127,* 585–586, 1958.

FREEMAN, R.D., MITCHELL, D.E., MOLLODOT, M.: A neural effect of partial visual deprivation in humans. Sci. *175,* 1384–1386, 1972.

FULLER, J.L.: Experimental deprivation and later behavior. Sci. *158,* 1645–1652, 1967.

GLOBUS, A., SCHEIBEL, A.B.: The effect of visual deprivation on cortical neurons: A Golgi study. Exper.Neurol. *19,* 331–345, 1967.

GREENOUGH, W.T.: The Nature and Nurture of Behavior. Readings from Scientific American. W.H.Freeman Co., 1973.

HARLOW, H.F.: Learning to Love. Jason Aronson, N.Y., 1974.

HELD, R., BAUER, J.A., Jr.: Visually guided reaching in infant monkeys after restricted rearing. Sci. *155,* 718–720, 1967.

HIRSCH, H.V.B., SPINELLI, D.N.: Visual experience modifies distribution of horizontally and vertically oriented receptive fields in cats. Sci. *168,* 869–871, 1970.

KARLSSON, J.-O., SJOSTRAND, J.: Effect of deprivation of light on axonal transport in retinal ganglion cells of the rabbit. Br.Res. *29,* 315–332, 1971.

LEVITSKY, D.A., BARNES, R.H.: Nutritional and environmental interactions in the behavioral development of the rat: long-term effects. Sci. *176,* 68–71, 1972.

LUND, R.D.: Development and Plasticity of the Brain. Oxford Univ.Press, N.Y., 1978.

MALETTA, G.J., TIMIRAS, P.S.: Acetylocholinesterase activity in optic structures after complete light deprivation from birth. Exper.Neurol. *19,* 513–518, 1967.

MELZACK, R.: Effects of early perceptual restriction on simple visual discrimination. Sci. *137,* 978–979, 1962.

NEVILLE, H.E., CHASE, H.P.: Undernutrition and cerebellar development. Exper.Neurol. *33,* 485–497, 1971.

PETTIGREW, J.E., FREEMAN, R.D.: Visual experience without lines: Effect on developing cortical neurons. Sci. *182,* 599–600, 1973.

RIESEN, A.H. (Ed.): The Developmental Neuropsychology of Sensory Deprivation. Academic Press, 1975.

RIZZOLATTI, G., TRADARDI, V.: Pattern discrimination in monocularly reared cats. Exper.Neurol. *33,* 181–194, 1971.

ROSENZWEIG, M.R., BENNET, E.L., DIAMOND, M.C., WU, S.Y., SLAGLE, R.W., SAFFRAN, E.: Influences of environmental complexity and visual stimulation on development of occipital cortex in rat. Br.Res. *14,* 427–445, 1969.

SACKETT, G.P.: Monkeys reared in isolation with pictures as visual input: Evidence for an innate releasing mechanism. Sci. *154,* 1468–1473, 1966.

SHERMAN, S.M.: Development of interocular alignment in cats. Br.Res. *37,* 187–203, 1972.

SHERMAN, S.M.: Visual field defects in monocularly and binocularly deprived cats. Br.Res. *49,* 25–45, 1973.

SHERMAN, S., SANDERSON, K.J.: Binocular interaction on cells of the dorsal lateral geniculate nucleus of visually deprived cats. Br.Res. *37,* 126–131, 1972.

SHLAER, R.: Shift in binocular disparity causes compensatory change in the cortical structure of kittens. Sci. *173,* 638–641, 1971.

VALVERDE, F.: Rate and extent of recovery from dark rearing in the visual cortex of the mouse. Br.Res. *33,* 1–11, 1971.

VANDERLOOS, H., WOOLSEY, T.A.: Somatosensory cortex: Structural alterations following early injury to sense organs. Sci. *179,* 395–397, 1973.

WENDT, R.H., LINDSLEY, D.F., ADEY, W.R., FOX, S.S.: Self-maintained visual stimulation in monkeys after long-term visual deprivation. Sci. *139,* 336–338, 1962.

WHITE, B.L.: The First Three Years of Life. Prentice-Hall, 1975.

Bibliography

1 ABRAHAMS, V.C.: The physiology of neck muscles: their role in head movement and maintenance of posture. Can.Jrl.Physiol. & Pharmacol. *55* (3), 332–338, 1977.

2 ABRAHAMS, V.C., RANCIER, F., ROSE, P.K.: Neck muscles and extraocular receptors and their relationship to the tectospinal tract. In: Stein, R.B., Pearon, K.B., Smith, R.S., Redford, J.B. (Eds.): Control of Posture and Locomotion. Plenum Publ.Corp. 1974.

3 ABRAHAMS, V.C., RICHMOND, F., ROSE, P.K.: Basic physiology of the head-eye movement system. In: Lennerstrand, G., Bach-y-Rita, P. (Eds.): Basic Mechanisms of Ocular Motility and Their Clinical Implications. Pergamon Press, 1975.

4 ABRAHAMS, V.C., RICHMOND, R., ROSE, P.K.: Absence of monosynaptic reflex in dorsal neck muscles of the cat. Br.Res. *92,* 130–131, 1975.

5 ALTMAN, J., DAS, G.D.: Autoradiographic examination of the effects of enriched environment on the rate of glial multiplication in the adult rat brain. Nature, 1161–1163, 1964.

6 ANNIS, R.C., FROST, B.: Human visual ecology and orientation anisotropies in acuity. Sci. *182,* 729–731, 1973.

7 ARUTIUNIAN, R.S.: Effect of vibration on receptors of fast and slow muscles. Fiziology Zh.S.S.S.R. *57,* 1298–1306, 1971.

8 BACH-Y-RITA, P.: Brain Mechanisms in Sensory Substitution. Academic Press, N.Y., 1972. p.192.

9 BARR, M.L.: The Human Nervous System, 2nd ed. Harper & Row, 1974.

10 BENNETT, E.L., DIAMOND, M.C., KRECH, D., ROSENZWEIG, M.R.: Chemical and anatomical plasticity of brain. Sci. *146,* 610–619, 1964.

11 BLAKEMORE, C.: Mechanics of the Mind. Cambridge Univ.Press, 1977.

12 BOWER, T.G.R.: Repetitive processes in child development. Sci.Am. 38–47, Nov. 1976.

13 BRIDGEMAN, E., ELDRED, E.: Hypothesis for a pressure-sensitive mechanism in muscle spindles. Sci. *143,* 481–482, 1964.

14 BRODAL, A.: Self-observations and neuro-anatomical considerations after a stroke. Brain *96,* 675–694, 1973.

15 BROWN, M.D., ENGBERG, I., MATTHEWS, P.B.C.: The relative sensitivity to vibration of muscle receptors of the cat. Jrl.Physiol. *192,* 773–800, 1967.

16 CHUSID, J.G.: Correlative Neuroanatomy and Functional Neurology. 15th ed. Lange Medical Pub., 1973.

17 CRAGG, B.G.: Changes in visual cortex on first exposure of rats to light. Nature *215,* 251–253, 1967.

18 CROSBY, E.C., HUMPHREY, T., LAUER, E.W.: Correlative Anatomy of the Nervous System. The MacMillan Company, 1962.

19 DIMOND, S.J., BLIZARD, D.A. (Eds.): Evolution and Lateralization of the Brain. N.Y. Acad.Sci. 1977.

20 ECCLES, J.C.: The Understanding of the Brain, 2nd ed. McGraw-Hill Book Company, N.Y., 1977.

21 FERCHMIN, P.A., ETEROVIC, V.A., CAPUTTO, R.: Studies of brain weight and RNA content after short period of exposure to environmental complexity. Br.Res. *20,* 49–57, 1970.

22 GRADY, A., GILFOYLE, E., MOORE, J.C.: Children Adapt. To be published by Charles Slack, Assoc. 1979.

23 GRANIT, R.: The Purposive Brain. MIT Press, Cambridge, Mass., 1977.

24 GREENOUGH, W.T.: The Nature and Nurture of Behavior. Readings from Scientific American. W.H.Freeman Co., 1973.

25 GUTH, L.: Axonal regeneration and functional plasticity in the central nervous system. Exper.Neurol. *45,* 606–654, 1974.

26 HELD, R.: Plasticity in sensory-motor systems. Sci.Am. 84–94, Nov. 1965.

27 HELD, R., FREEDMAN, S.J.: Plasticity in human sensorimotor control. Sci. *142,* 455–462, 1963.

28 HOLLOWAY, R.L., Jr.: Dendritic branching: Some preliminary results of training and complexity in rat visual cortex. Br.Res. *2,* 393–396, 1966.

29 HORN, G., ROSE, S.R.F., BATESON, P.P.G.: Experience and plasticity in the central nervous system. Sci. *181,* 506–514, 1973.

30 HORRIDGE, G.A.: Mechanistic teleology and explanation in neuroethology. Bio.Sci. 27 (11), 725–732, 1977.

31 LEMIRE, R.J., LOESER, J.D., LEECH, R.W., ALVORD, E.C., Jr.: Normal and Abnormal Development of the Human Nervous System. Harper and Row, 1975.

32 LIPTON, M.A.: Early experience and plasticity in the central nervous system. In: Tjossem, T.D. (Ed.): Intervention Strategies for High Risk Infants and Young Children. Univ.Park Press, 1976.

33 LURIA, A.R.: Higher Cortical Functions in Man. Basic Books, 1966.

34 MOORE, J.C.: Concepts From the Neurobehavioral Sciences. Kendall/Hunt Pub., Dubuque, 1973.

35 MOORE, K.L.: The Developing Human. W.B. Saunders, 1974.

36 PAINE, R.S., BRAZELTON, T.B., DONOVAN, D.E., DRORBAUGH, J.E., HUBBELL, J.P., SEARS, E.M.: Evolution of postural reflexes in normal infants and in the presence of chronic brain syndromes. Jrl. Neurology 11, 1036–1048, 1964.

37 PEELE, T.L.: The Neuroanatomical Basis for Clinical Neurology, 3rd ed. McGraw-Hill, Inc., 1977.

38 PEIPER, A.: Cerebral Function in Infancy and Childhood. Consultants Bureau, New York, 1963.

39 RAISMAN, G.: Neuronal plasticity in the septal nuclei of the adult rat. Br. Res. 14, 25–48, 1969.

40 RAISMAN, G.: Electron microscopic studies of the development of new neurohaemal contacts in the median eminence of the rat after hypophysectomy. Br.Res. 55, 245–261, 1973.

41 RAISMAN, G., FIELD, P.M.: A quantitative investigation of the development of collateral reinnervation after partial diafferentation of the septal nuclei. Br.Res. 50, 241–264, 1973.

42 RICHMOND, F.J.R., ABRAHAMS, V.C.: Morphology and distribution of muscle spindles in dorsal muscles of the cat neck. Jrl.Neurophysiol. 58 (6) 1322–1330, 1975.

43 RICHMOND, F.J.R., ABRAHAMS, V.C.: Morphology and enzyme histochemistry of dorsal muscles of the cat neck. Jrl.Neurophysiol. 38 (6), 1312–1321, 1975.

44 RUTLEDGE, L.T., DUNCAN, J., BEATTY, N.: A study of pryamidal cell axon collaterals in intact and partially isolated adult cerebral cortex. Br. Res. 16, 15–22, 1969.

45 SARNAT, H.B., NETSKY, M.G.: Evolution of the Nervous System. Oxford Univ.Press, 1974.

46 SATO, M.: Response of pacinian corpuscles to sinusoidal vibration. Jrl. Physiol. 159, 391–409, 1961.

47 SHERRINGTON, C.: The Integrative Action of the Nervous System. New Haven Univ.Press, 1961.

48 STEIN, D., ROSEN, J.J., BUTTERS, N. (Eds.): Plasticity and Recovery of Function in the Central Nervous System. Academic Press, 1974.

49 TROTT, J.R.: Reflex responses of fusimotor neurones during muscle vibration. J.Physiol. (London) 247 (1) 20P–22P, 1975.

50 TUCHMANN-DUPLESSIS, H., AUROUX, M., HAEGEL, P.: Illustrated Human Embryology, Vol.III, Nervous System and Endocrine Glands, Springer, N.Y., 1975.

51 URBSCHEIT, N., BISHOP, B.: Effects of cooling on the ankle jerk and H-response. Phys.Ther. *50* (7), 1041–1049, July, 1970.

52 VOLKMAR, F.R., GREENOUGH, W.T.: Rearing complexity affects branching of dendrites in the visual cortex of the rat. Sci. *176,* 1445–1447, 1972.

53 WALL, P.D., EGGER, M.D.: Formation of new connections in adult rat brains after partial deafferentation. Nature *232,* 542–545, 1971.

54 WILLIAMS and WARWICK: Functional Neuroanatomy of Man, W.B. Saunders Co., 1975.

55 WILLIS, W.D., Jr., GROSSMAN, R.G.: Medical Neurobiology, 2nd ed. C.V. Mosby Co., 1977.

Mechanisms of plasticity of connection following damage in adult mammalian nervous systems

PATRICK D. WALL

The Problem: There is no doubt in the mind of any clinician that reparative processes must exist in the brain of adults. Sudden destruction of brain or spinal cord by vascular accident, by gun shot or by neurosurgery is followed immediately by the worst signs and symptoms which the patient will exhibit. With survival, there is some amelioration of the initial signs. What are the mechanisms of this recovery process? In addition to the existence of recovery, we must take into account at least two crucial aspects of the process. The first is that it is slow. Some changes may occur within hours but the final plateau level of recovery will not be achieved for months. The second aspect we must include in any explanation is related to the first; slow destruction of brain tissue has less severe consequences than a sudden production of the same amount of destruction. This is seen in slowly growing tumours, when the patient's first signs and symptoms may first present at a time when a huge area of brain has been destroyed. Immediate destruction of the same volume of brain would produce devastating signs whereas the tumour patients often present with trivial signs or with secondary signs such as epilepsy or increased intracranial pressure. This effect has been seen repeatedly in experimental animals where spaced neurosurgical partial excisions of an area of cortex leading to complete removal produce minor changes when compared to complete removal of the area at a single session. It is evident then that some recovery process exists with a relatively slow time course and with some limitation on its maximal extent.

Solutions to the problem

1) Partial secondary solutions

There are certain changes which undoubtedly contribute to recovery but which should not divert us from the main problem. Any disease or damage will have a threshold for permanent destruction. Even a surgical lesion has an edge in which cells will be temporarily incapacitated by trauma. The extreme example is a toxic encephalopathy where recovery will occur if the toxin can be reduced below its effective level. The spectacular recoveries which can occur after a virus encephalitis may well be explained by the temporary inactivation of neurons during the height of the virus invasion. Nerve cells do not suddenly change from normal full activity to irreversible death. The intermediate recoverable reversible states undoubtedly explain some parts of the recovery process. One is most tempted to use this as an explanation in the case of vascular disease. If a cerebral artery is suddenly occluded, there will be an area of brain which undergoes irreversible ischaemic damage and necrosis. Necessarily there will be an edge to this zone, where cells will survive with a relatively intact morphology because they retain a partial blood supply which is not sufficient to allow normal function. This edge containing surviving but inactive cells may be slowly invaded by new capillaries which re-establish sufficient blood supply to allow a return of function to the sleeping but asphyxiated princesses. This may well be a real and important process but we must not forget the pathology which is found in the brains of patients who have made a nearly complete recovery from strokes. This shows considerable total loss of brain tissue in certain areas. This loss may be crudely measured by a decrease of overall brain weight or by more subtle measures such as arteriography showing the retention of minimally circulated areas or by CAT scans showing areas with a grossly abnormal morphology or by histology showing scarred areas containing only the debris of formerly highly organized regions of brain. These areas of total and permanent destruction are so great and so frequently discovered that we cannot attribute the recovery of the stroke victim to the recovery of brain areas which have been permanently destroyed.

A violent episode in the brain will trigger local and reflex changes of the vasculature and of the ionic environment around nerve cells. Concussion is an example of the latter where sudden movement triggers a wave of spreading depression across the whole area. This state is not accompanied by gross morphological change and lasts considerably less than one hour. Reflex and locally propagated changes in the vasculature following trauma certainly occur. They can be directly observed under experimental conditions. However we cannot use these changes to explain the long term and long distance changes which are observed during recovery. Traumatic paraplegia is a good example of this because here we have locally damaged spinal cord supplied by its local segmental arteries and yet changes of excitability occur in very distant segments over periods of weeks and months. If a clean transection of the spinal cord in the upper thoracic region occurs, there will be, of course, an immediate commotion of the entire autonomic system and there will be local and general changes of the vasculature. In an uncomplicated case, there is no evidence of any distant area of ischaemia after a few hours or days and yet it is just at this time that the expected progress of changes of reflex excitability in the isolated cord begin to occur and will proceed for months until the final permanent chronic state is established. Therefore, we must consider vascular and metabolic changes as playing a crucial role during the acute stages immediately following damage to the central nervous system. However in the days, weeks and months after the event, these changes are highly unlikely to be crucial. If anyone still wishes to maintain that these are the effective controls of recovery, they must provide experimental evidence for their hypotheses. This is not an unreasonable requirement since there are many accurate quantitative measures of regional blood flow, biochemical concentrations and metabolic activity. The availability of these experimental methods means that experiments can be designed to check to see if the cardiovascular and metabolic changes which follow a lesion can be shown to be correlated with functional recovery. So far such correlations have not been shown.

2) Forbidden solutions

When tissue such as liver or kidney or skin is damaged, recovery occurs by mitotic duplication of cells. The new cells migrate and differentiate into newly functioning cells. There is no evidence that this process occurs in adult brain.

When peripheral nerve is cut across, the axons separated from their cell bodies degenerate. The central cut end of the axon then emits sprouts, some of which may grow along the distal Schwann cells and may reach the original destination of the nerve fibre. In the central nervous system, the same degeneration occurs, sprouts are emitted but the necessary medium for long range growth of the sprouts does not exist. Therefore regeneration as is known in the periphery does not occur in the C.N.S. There are always some signs of local sprouting and even of establishment of contacts with nearby cells which have lost their afferent axons as a result of the injury. These new local contacts are frequently anatomically incorrect in that the original input is lost and replaced by the sprout of a nearby axon which has no relevant message for the cell. Thus there is no evidence for successful useful regeneration of cut axons in brain or spinal cord.

Just as we have said that cells may be temporarily partially reversibly damaged, this may also occur with axons. A local anaesthetic temporarily blocks conduction. More seriously, simple demyelination may leave a bare axon capable of occasional and low frequency transmission. Such conduction is fragile and easily influenced by small changes of the immediate environment. This state may explain the rapid transient variability of diseases such as multiple sclerosis. A more permanent restoration of function can occur with remyelination of the stripped axons. However, this process cannot explain recovery where frank destruction of the axons has occurred.

3) Mystical solutions

The neurological literature is full of words which imply understanding but which only describe the process they are purported to explain. The smart medical student knows that the answer to the question, «Why can a patient not remember the circumstances of his head injury?» is «Because the patient has post-traumatic amnesia». He has been taught that nomination is explanation. Quite serious textbooks state that the early areflexic state of paraplegia is caused by spinal shock. «Spinal shock» is not a cause of anything, it is a circular confusing description of the state of areflexia. Furthermore, at a later stage, the paraplegic is not recovering from spinal shock, he is in fact recovering. Shock, diaschisis, disorganisation etc. are examples of obfuscating words which imply understanding but actually submerge ignorance of mechanism.

I find that the word «redundancy» approaches mysticism in its use to explain recovery. The implication of the word is that there exist systems of alternative circuits in the brain which can be switched on when one system fails. We almost never read any details of what these alternate systems could be. Obviously they could come in two classes. One class would be where there is an exact duplication implying that the system is overbuilt in the embryo. It is frequently suggested that peripheral sensory nerves represent such a class of excess. The evidence is that a peripheral nerve can be slowly destroyed in a disease such as leprosy and that destruction must proceed to over 50% before clinical signs appear. I think this is very weak evidence. Our clinical tests measure only a basic minimum of performance and never push the system to exhibit its maximum possibilities of simultaneous transmission of different types of information. There are of course systems which are strictly duplicated, eye, ears, and hands. A visitor from outer space might initially believe that these were redundant structures until deeper study would show that duplication allowed special functions to evolve. I do not believe that we can declare redundancy of identical duplicated structures on the basis of tests which measure isolated simple functions of systems clearly capable of sophisticated analysis.

The second use of the word redundancy suggests that alternative systems with different workings can carry out the same functional role. On a crude level this is obviously true. A man may «walk» in the ordinary way, or, if he has paralysed legs, he may «walk» using his abdomical muscles to tilt and swing his pelvis. A blind man may «navigate» using his non-visual systems. No-one would suggest that these alternative mechanisms mean that they are redundant in the normal man and yet this is exactly the argument used to explain the lack of symptomatology associated with brain lesions. I have written elsewhere on this topic using the dorsal columns as an example (WALL [13, 14]). If the dorsal columns are cut across, the classical dorsal column signs do not appear. That is to say man and animals are capable of feeling and locating light touch and vibration and of identifying texture and weight. The explanation that has been given is that there are redundant systems available either of which are capable of transmitting the necessary information so that if the main system is lost then the other takes over its function. We have shown that this conclusion is fundamentally wrong and again comes from the use of exceedingly simple tests which fail to challenge the full capability of the system. We found that while no single modality is lost as a result of dorsal column lesions there is a permanent loss of the ability to analyse simultaneously the spatial and temporal characteristics of the stimulus (WALL & NOORDENBOS [16]).

4) Permissable solutions

What then are the mechanisms which are known to exist in brain which could be used to explain the observed recovery.

A. Learning alternative strategies

I will mention this only briefly since it is the most obvious factor and the basis of much of rehabilitation medicine. If a man loses his dominant right hand, he is taught and learns to improve the skill of his left and to substitute one handed for bimanual tasks. If a patient becomes blind, he is taught and learns to use subtle cues from his other senses which previously existed but had been ignored. We know nothing of the mechanisms by which motor and sensory skills are developed.

96

However important this mechanism may be, it is quite clear that some other inexorable process is in operation by which the patient regains motor and sensory abilities almost in spite of his and his therapists efforts.

B. *Sprouting of intact axons*

We have said that adult mammalian central axons when cut across fail to regenerate. This leaves their terminal synaptic regions empty. In some manner, nearby intact axons sense the presence of these evacuated synaptic sites, send out sprouts and occupy them. This process has been best studied in the periphery where partial denervation of muscle is followed by the sprouting of intact motor axons which send out sprouts which occupy and excite the motor end plates which have been vacated by the degeneration of their former axons (EDDS [7]). Not all peripheral axons are capable of such collateral sprouting. The preganglionic axons from spinal cord to sympathetic ganglia do not occupy vacated sites in the ganglion. It seems that these fibres have grown to their maximal size in the embryo and are incapable of expanding their terminal field.

In the central nervous system there is clear evidence that collateral sprouting occurs. RAISMAN and FIELD [11] have studied cells in adult rat septal nuclei. These cells receive inputs originating from two separate areas. If either of these areas are destroyed, the other input spreads to occupy the entire surface of the cell body and dendrites formerly shared by the two inputs. It is not known how far these sprouts can reach and the evidence at the moment suggests that they grow only very short distances perhaps less than 1 mm.

One must ask if collateral sprouting is advantageous and if it promotes recovery. In the case of partially denervated muscle, one can easily see that there is a powerful advantage. Muscle fibres which would otherwise contribute nothing to the strength of muscle contraction are recruited back to contraction by expansion of the number of muscle fibres innervated by a single motor axon. There will be a slight loss of graded control of contraction since fewer axons are involved but this is a small price to pay for the return of muscle strength. However this recovery comes from the fact that all of the motor axons to a single muscle were contributing to the same task and were therefore equivalent. Turning to the central nervous system, it will readily be understood that equivalence of task of neighbouring axons is rare. Different types of axon converge on cells bringing in different types of information and control. If one type is lost by a destructive lesion and the survivors expanded to occupy empty sites, the cell may now regain a highly abnormal function. Furthermore the occupation of empty sites may be one of the factors preventing successful regeneration of the cut axons. It will be seen that the retention of the embryonic ability to form nerve sprouts may be a double edged sword either capable of restoring partial restoration of function or of introducing abnormal or useless or disadvantageous function. We need to know the functional rules of collateral sprouting. If there is a recapitulation of embryonic development where only certain ordered contacts can be made, the cell may regain some of its previous role. However, if there is a simple rush by the nearest axons to occupy evacuated territory then there may be no advantage or a positive disadvantage.

C. Modulation of existing axons and synapses

Here we ask a question about whether existing synapses which are not destroyed by a lesion can be brought into action. Is there a background in the brain of anatomically established synapses which can be called upon when the usually dominating systems fail. There are two quite different series of experiments which suggest that this may be the case.

1) What is the effect of activity on synaptic transmission?

A homeostatic mechanism might exist where a decrease of input activity would be followed by an increase in excitability. The effect of this adjustment would be that a partial loss of input would produce a compensation so that the remaining input would have a larger effect. I would like to draw attention to an old elegant series of experiments reviewed by SPENCER and APRIL which suggest that just such a process is in operation (SPENCER & APRIL [12]). They simply cut the Achilles tendon in adult cats and also cut the ventral roots which supplied the gastrocnemius. An effect of this operation is to decrease the afferent barrage originating from the spindles in the muscle. A major central target in the spinal cord of these afferent impulses is Clarke's column. Their experiments show that increased synaptic effectiveness of the group 1 afferent fibres is associated with the chronic disuse of the afferents. This conclusion came from stimulation of the sensory afferents from the silenced muscle and recording of the discharge from the cells in Clarke's column. The size of the evoked afferent sensory volley was exactly the same from the used and the disused muscle. The size of the response from the nucleus whose afferents had been relatively silent was much larger than the response from the nucleus whose afferents had carried the usual ongoing afferent barrage. The authors attribute the increased excitability of the nucleus to the lowered impulse traffic over the afferents. One should not forget that tenotomy and the cutting of the ventral roots will produce marked morphological changes in the muscle. This may produce changes of the sensory axons and certainly may change the amount and nature of substances transported along the afferent axons to the nucleus. However, whether the changes are produced by decreased impulse traffic or by morphological change or by a change of transported substances, the effect of a compensatory increase of excitability could be of considerable interest in recovery processes.

2) What is the effect of partial deafferentation

In a large series of experiments recently reviewed (MERRILL & WALL [9]), we have observed the effects of partial destruction of the afferent input to a region. This has been done in adult rat thalamus by removal of one nucleus of the dorsal column nuclei (WALL & EGGER [15]). This was followed over days and weeks by a gradual expansion of the innervated zone into the denervated zone. Similar types of experiments were carried out in adult cat by sectioning of dorsal roots followed by examination of the denervated zones of dorsal column nuclei and of the spinal cord (BASBAUM & WALL [1], MILLAR, BASBAUM & WALL [10], DOSTROVSKY, MILLAR & WALL [6]). In each situation we found that cells which had lost their input began to respond to intact afferents. In the dorsal column nuclei we found a special class of cell which instantly switched their input immediately on the silencing of their normal input. We could silence the input reversibly by cold block and here we saw the receptive fields immediately switched back and forth from one location to another widely separated location. Clearly in this case some ongoing physiological activity was holding one input pathway suppressed. As soon as the major input failed, the inhibition of the alternative input failed revealing this new excitatory pathway. However, this immediate switching mechanism was never seen in spinal cord and did not apply to the bulk of the dorsal column nucleus cells which eventually changed their receptive fields. For the majority of cells the change took days and weeks to complete the full appearance of the new receptive field in its full state of excitability.

What could be the explanation of these slow changes of receptive field? Could they be due to sprouting or could they be some unmasking of existing connections. To entertain the latter possibility we have to show that suitable afferents actually exist. We have shown that sensory fibres entering the dorsal root terminate in the cord not only in the immediate vicinity of the entry segment but also send long ranging axons which extend over many segments rostral and caudal to the entry root (WALL & WERMAN [17]). Physiological studies using natural peripheral stimuli show no cells responding to these distant afferents in the intact animal. If electrical stimuli are used which have a particularly efficient central excitatory effect because of the synchronisation of the arriving volley, small numbers of distant cells are discovered responding to the long range afferents (DEVOR, MERRILL & WALL [5]). If however roots close to the recorded cells are destroyed then very large numbers of cells respond to the long range afferents when either electrical or natural stimuli are used (BASBAUM &

WALL [1]). Therefore, there are afferents present which provide a potential source of new input in the presence of degeneration.

We are left with the question of mechanism by which normally ineffective inputs become effective. It was possible in the presence of degeneration that the degeneration of afferents induced sprouting of intact afferents which occupied the vacated sites. On the other hand there could be a slow transynaptic degeneration of inhibitory mechanisms which unmask the activity of anatomically existing contacts. We were unable to resolve this question by this type of experiment and therefore changed to a new type which has produced a surprising and clear cut effect.

3) What is the effect of cutting peripheral nerve fibres on the connectivity of spinal cord cells?

When peripheral nerves are cut, the spinal cord cells no longer receive their normal afferent barrage and substances transported from the periphery do not arrive. However, there is no gross anatomical degeneration and therefore synaptic sites are not vacated.

The dorsal horn of lumbar segments 6 and 7 in adult cat cord contain somatotopically organised cells with the foot and toes represented medially and the upper and lower leg laterally (BROWN & FUCHS [2]). If the sciatic and saphenous nerves are cut, in mid thigh, the foot and toes become completely anaesthetic. We cut these nerves in one leg of adult cats and allowed them to recover for various periods of time (DEVOR & WALL [4]). Then on the observation day, the animal was anaesthetised, decerebrated and the spinal cord transected at L1. This preparation in our experience produces a lumbar spinal cord with very lively response to cutaneous peripheral stimulation. In the experimental leg, the sciatic and saphenous nerves were exposed again and resectioned proximal to the original cut. This was done to eliminate any possible sprouts which might have grown out of the sectioned end. Next on the intact leg, the sciatic and saphenous nerves were sectioned on the experimental day. This allowed the spinal cord to be examined where one side has been chronically de-afferented in comparison to the other side which had suffered the identical deafferentation on the experimental day. The deafferented dorsal horns were searched for single cells responding to natural stimuli of the legs. In each animal, the dorsal horn was searched to a depth of 2 mm below the surface with a series of parallel tracks separated by 100 μm beginning at the midline and moving laterally to beyond the dorsal root entry zone (REZ). Sixteen maps were completed in 12 cats with acutely deafferented dorsal horns with a total of 156 search tracks at or medial to the REZ. In all animals a cluster of cells was located in the dorsolateral gray matter with receptive fields (RFs) on the upper and lower leg. These cells and their response characteristics appeared identical to those described in the intact cat (DEVOR & WALL [4]). As penetrations moved more than 200 μm medial to the REZ, large numbers of cells were encountered which have ongoing activity but which failed to respond to peripheral stimulation. In this medial area, we located only 8 responding cells in 108 search tracks. All 8 required pressure on the upper or lower leg to excite them. In the intact cat, virtually all cells in this region respond to brush, touch or pressure stimuli on foot or toes.

We examined 7 animals who had survived 28–105 days after nerve section on one side. The most obvious change was that the most medial track containing responding cells had moved from about 200 μm medial to the REZ on the acutely deafferented side to the far medial edge of the dorsal horn. All told, in 69 dorsal horn tracks more than 200 μm medial to the REZ, 94% (65 tracks) contained cells with RFs on the legs versus 7% in the acutely deafferented cords. Many of the cells responded to brush or touch. The size, nature and position of the RFs covered the same range as those previously described for laterally placed cells with proximal RFs in intact animals and as those we observed here in the same region in the acutely deafferented dorsal horns. The latency of the fastest response to electrical stimulation applied to the RF was measured for 99 medial cells. The distribution of these latencies was similar to that of the laterally located cells with proximal RFs seen in intact and acutely deafferented cats. It extended from 2.5–15 msec. Those cells responding in 2.5–4 msec may be considered good candidates for having a monosynaptic contact with afferents and they made up 19% of the population. The change in dorsal horn connectivity appeared fully developed by 28 days. In experiments on animals with shorter survival times signs are apparent that the change has begun as early as 6 days after peripheral nerve section.

While it is true that many cells remained without peripheral RFs even in the longest surviving animals, it is apparent that large numbers of cells in a region of cord normally dominated by afferents from foot and toes begin to respond to other areas of the leg some days or weeks after section of the peripheral axons which previously supplied their excitatory drive. The new RFs found in the former toe-foot region are all in skin supplied by remaining intact cutaneous nerves.

What changes centrally after peripheral nerve section that could account for this shift? We could detect no signs of degeneration among the central terminals of the afferents whose periphery had been cut. There was no gross atrophy of the dorsal horn. Therefore we must presume that, unlike the situation after dorsal root section, there could be no marked morphological changes in the cord. One would guess that this situation would not allow sprouting to establish new contacts. However, it is possible that small readjustments of contact could take place with atrophy of some boutons and expansion of others. Some such subtle changes have been seen in the substantia gelatinosa after section of peripheral nerves. It would seem that the signal for shift of connection is most likely to be either the change of the arriving impulse traffic or of the substances transported into spinal cord over dorsal roots from the periphery.

Summary and conclusions

We began with the fact that those who survive brain damage show a surprising degree of recovery. No doubt some of this recovery is to be attributed to readjustments of blood vessels and other factors on which the brain depends. However some degree of recovery is seen even where there is known permanent destruction of parts of the central nervous system. Certain mechanisms cannot be proposed to explain this recovery. Brain cells in the adult do not divide to produce new cells. Nerve fibres cut across in the central nervous system do not regenerate as they do in the periphery. Certain suggestions to explain recovery are rejected as being unhelpful and mystical since they do not specify what it is that has changed during recovery. Words such as shock, diaschisis and redundancy are not useful. There is no doubt that the patient learns to substitute alternative mechanisms for those he has lost just as a blind man develops his skills of hearing and feeling and just as an amputee extends the repertoire of his remaining limbs. Beyond this crucial learning there are signs of unlearned readjustments within the brain. Nerve cells show a type of homeostasis so that if they lose part of their input, they adjust their excitability to capture fully the excitatory effects of their remaining input. When nerve fibres degenerate, the nearby intact fibres have an ability to sprout and occupy the sites left vacant by the degenerated fibres. Beyond this sprouting mechanism there are large numbers of normally ineffective nerve connections which may become active if the dominant inputs are put out of action. It is proposed that the connections laid down in the embryo are more diffuse than those actually used in the adult brain. The stage of maturation involves partly destruction of the «incorrect» connections and partly their suppression. If some nervous connections are destroyed in the adult, suppressed connections may become derepressed. This process is not necessarily a good thing, the substituted connections may bring in nonsense information which the recovering nervous system cannot handle. Sprouting and the unmasking of ineffective connections offers the possibility of new connections after brain damage but we need to know much more about these processes so that we can guide them to useful ends rather than towards further disorganisation.

Bibliography

1 BASBAUM, A., WALL, P.D.: Chronic changes in the response of cells in adult cat dorsal horn following partial deafferentation. Brain Res. *116,* 181–204, 1976.

2 BROWN, P.B., FUCHS, J.L.: Somatotopic representation of hind limb skin in cat dorsal horn. J.Neurophysiol. *38,* 1–9, 1975.

3 DEVOR, M., MERRILL, E.G., WALL, P.D.: Dorsal horn cells that respond to stimulation of distant dorsal roots. J.Physiol. *270,* 519–531, 1977.

4 DEVOR, M., WALL, P.D.: Dorsal horn cells with proximal cutaneous receptive fields. Brain Res. *118,* 325–328, 1976.

5 DEVOR, M., WALL, P.D.: Reorganisation of the spinal cord's sensory map after peripheral nerve injury. Nature (in press).

6 DOSTROVSKY, J.O., MILLAR, J., WALL, P.D.: The immediate shift of afferent drive of dorsal column nucleus cells following deafferentation. Exp.Neurol. *52,* 480–495, 1976.

7 EDDS, M.V.: Collateral nerve regeneration. Quart.Rev.Biol. *28,* 260–276, 1953.

8 KNYIHAR, E., CSILLIK, B.: Effect of peripheral axotomy on the fine structure of the Rolando substance. Exp.Brain Res. *26,* 73–87, 1976.

9 MERRILL, E.G., WALL, P.D.: Plasticity of connection in the adult nervous system. In: Cotman, C.W. (Ed.): Neuronal plasticity. New York, Raven Press, 1978; pp.97–111.

10 MILLAR, J., BASBAUM, A.I., WALL, P.D.: Restructuring of the somatotopic map and appearance of abnormal neuronal activity in the gracile nucleus after partial deafferentation. Exp.Neurol. *50,* 658–672, 1976.

11 RAISMAN, G., FIELD, P.M.: A quantitative investigation of the development of collateral reinnervation of the septal nuclei. Brain Res. *50,* 241–264, 1973.

12 SPENCER, W.A., APRIL, R.S.: Plastic properties of monosynaptic pathways in mammals. In: Horn, G., Hinde, R.A. (Eds.): Short term changes in neural activity and behaviour. London, Cambridge University Press, 1970; pp.433–473.

13 WALL, P.D.: The sensory and motor role of impulses travelling in the dorsal columns toward the cerebral cortex. Brain *93,* 505–524, 1970.

14 WALL, P.D.: The somatosensory system. In: Gazzaniga, M.S., Blakemore, C. (Eds.): Handbook of psychobiology. New York, Academic Press, 1975; pp.373–392.

15 WALL, P.D., EGGER, M.D.: Formation of new connections in adult rat brains after partial deafferentation. Nature *232,* 542–545, 1971.

16 WALL, P.D., NOORDENBOS, W.: Sensory functions which remain in man after complete transection of dorsal horns. Brain *100,* 641–653, 1978.

17 WALL, P.D., WERMAN, R.: The physiology and anatomy of long ranging afferent fibres within the spinal cord. J.Physiol. *255,* 321–334, 1976.

Functional cerebral reorganization following hemispherectomy in man and after small experimental lesions in primates

PAUL GLEES

Introduction

The study of recovery of brain function, the search for surviving or residual neural function following traumatic damage or surgical interference, is of utmost importance for a well directed program of rehabilitation. Only when the parameters of neurological dimensions of residual brain tissue are fully understood, can persisting and successful steps for the patient's integration in a restricted or normal environment be embarked upon. For these reasons, two aspects of my research experiences have been selected:

a) from human cases of hemispherectomy, the most drastic surgical intervention possible, leading to a varying direct loss of brain tissue from 170–300 g.

b) from experiments in primates recovering from selected removal of cerebral cortex in the motor and sensory areas.

Observations of both aspects show the remarkable ability of the remaining brain tissue for reorganization and the achievement of useful function for the total organism. The data presented here should therefore be looked upon mainly for the purpose of encouraging programs of rehabilitation and not so much for very detailed information on certain neurological topics, for which the quoted references should be consulted.

Three cases of hemispherectomy have been selected for this paper to emphasize that one hemisphere is sufficient to sustain a personality in locomotion, sensory perception of the whole body, speech and in a relatively normal social contact with his environment.

106

In order to get a better understanding of cerebral capabilities it will be necessary to look for the unexpected preservation of function or recovery of lost skill normally not to be hoped for or not even thought possible when taking a conventional view of cerebral pathways. Such a new source of information, unexpected and not conforming with traditional neural concepts, proved to be the study of cases of hemispherectomy.

Observations

Physiological and neuroanatomical observations of hemispherectomy were made while I was a research associate of the late Professor Sir HUGH CAIRNS, Radcliffe Infirmary, Oxford and at Göttingen University through the kind offices of Professor BUSHE, Department of Neurosurgery and Dr. H. BOEHNKE, Kinderkrankenhaus Hamburg. Not only was it possible to study cases before and after hemispherectomy, but I was also able to collect material for neuroanatomical studies and had the additional advantage of discussing some findings with Dr. D.H. OPPENHEIMER, the neuropathologist of the Radcliffe Infirmary, Oxford, whom I wish to thank here. Relevant questions, such as cerebral dominance, the function of the corpus callosum, what controls the residual motor power in the affected limbs, the evaluation of sensory data from one half of the body deprived of the receiving hemisphere, are of crucial importance to all problems of rehabilitation of patients deprived of brain tissue whether caused by injury or malformation. Concerning cerebral dominance and postoperative brain functions, one case (FABISCH et al., 1955) should be reviewed first in this context. The patient (DW) was extensively observed for a number of years. DW was operated on by the late Sir HUGH CAIRNS. This patient had a normal development until one year old and appeared to have a right hand preference. At the beginning of his second year, he had a series of fits and was admitted to the hospital. When discharged, a paralysis of the right arm and leg was noticed and his further mental development was initially delayed, but he was able to speak after a few weeks. After the age of two, fits started again, slowing down his development and causing difficulties at school, where his concentration was found to be poor. At the age of 10, he was sent to Lingfield Epileptic Colony where his fits, about once a month, continued. DW returned home when he was 16 years old, showing behavioral difficulties – a shortened dragging right leg, while the right arm was kept hanging straight down from the shoulder and swinging little when walking. The removal of the left hemisphere was carried out when the patient was 20 years old. Immediately after operation, right arm and leg were less spastic and the right arm was weaker than before operation. The distal part of the arm showed transient analgesia and anesthesia, but his ability for speech remained unimpaired. A week after operation, the patient showed voluntary movements of his right leg, but his motor ability of the right arm was reduced when compared with his preoperative condition. Sensory discrimination in the right leg, particularly proprioception, was very good, while position sense of the fingers of the right hand was inaccurate. He had a period, after operation, at Farnham Park Rehabilitation Center and regained partial use of his right hand (e.g., see Figure 2). There was then some delay in his training and placement, but eventually he was sent to St. Loyes College, Exeter, and trained for a year as a gardener. He worked first at a private house and then for the Nottingham Hospital for about nine months in all. This was his first attempt at remunerative work. He was considered too slow, and was rated as capable of only a tenth the capacity of mental patients employed in the gardens of the hospital. Despite discouragement, he joined the Y.M.C.A., learned basket work and dancing and took up photography. He came to Morris Motors, after being out of work for a year, following an approach by the hospital almoner in January 1956 and was placed in the Sheltered Workshop doing minor bench subassembly work. He settled down quickly, worked hard and mixed well with the other 50 disabled people – so much so that his supervisor asked for him to be taken on permanently (cf., GLEES & WHITE, 1958, and Figs. 1 and 2).

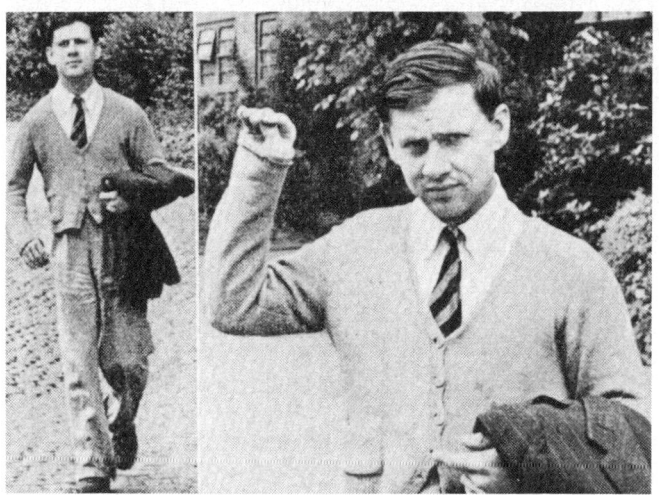

Figure 1. DW 3 years after hemispherectomy, walking freely and lifting his spastic hand on command.

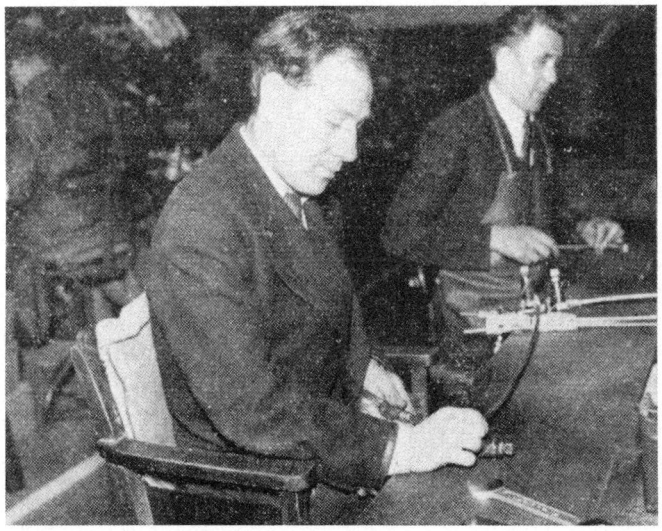

Figure 2. The same patient at work (Morris Motors, Oxford) using his right hand as well.

At an average, his day's work was as follows:

1) 100 trafficator switches
   (On this operation it is necessary to strip back the outer cover on the cable which is attached to the switch and snip off the surplus which is not required. Each switch has then to have about an inch of insulating tape applied.)

2) 288 number plate illumination lamps
   (This operation consists of removing the 2 B. A. nut with a box spanner; removing the cover, glass and the bulb; and putting the items into separate boxes for issue to the assembly lines.)

3) 3 only, heater control quadrants
   (This operation consists of attaching 1 inner and 2 outer control cables (similar to Bowden wire controls) and a box spanner is necessary for tightening six nuts, two of which are already attached.)

The patient had no fits since Christmas 1956 and his ouside interests include elementary photography, churchgoing and Bible reading. He had no girlfriends and, although he would have liked female company, he had a rather childish attitude towards such associations.

The second case (RL) had left spastic hemiplegia with severe attacks of epilepsy and suffered from aggressive behavior. He was unable to read or write at the age of 9. His right hemisphere, removed at the age of 10, showed severe cortical destruction of the central and inferior temporal areas and the region of the visual cortex (OPPENHEIMER & GRIFFITH, 1966). Together with Dr. W.G.WHITE, Chief Medical Officer at Morris Motors, Oxford, a careful study, including a film of his record and behavior, was made when he was accepted at the Sheltered Workshop six years after operation at the age of 16. While being observed, examined and filmed, he was friendly and cooperative, although of very childish behavior. During the period of observation, he was able to perform simple manual tasks, using his left hand as a prop. But he had voluntary movements of left arm and leg and some flexion of left thumb (Fig.3). Sensory perception of skin touch was delayed, pain localization inaccurate, but shape recognition in his left hand was fair. We found him much improved six years after operation when compared with his preoperative condition and he had learned to read and write in a slow cumbersome fashion.

However, at the age of 20, his physical and mental condition deteriorated progressively and he died at the age of 21. A detailed postmortem examination (OPPENHEIMER & GRIFFITH, 1966) showed superficial haemosiderosis of the central nervous system, chronic granular ependymitis, leading to obstruction of the C.S.F. pathways. Furthermore, he had multiple bleeding points in the membrane which had replaced the missing hemisphere and into the extension of this membrane into the lining of the ventricular system.

The third case (PG) which could be studied and filmed before and after operation in 1950, had his right hemisphere removed when he was 19 years old. The removed cerebral tissue amounted to 270 g. The patient had shown an epileptic fit at the age of 3½ years. The fits started in more severe form at the age of 10, when he had twitchings starting in the left arm and shoulder followed by the left leg. At the age of 14, the right arm area of the motor cortex was excised leading to a spastic left hemiplegia without abolishing his seizures, which were frequent and combined with severe confusion, absent-mindedness and dysphasia. After a right hemispheral removal, he lost his fits, felt well and made a remarkable recovery in mental faculties. He was able to obtain a university diploma and hold an administrative position. This patient was one of the most intelligent persons followed up among the 12 cases tested and compared by GRIFFITH & DAVIDSON (1966). On account of his friendly and cooperative personality after operation, I found him a valuable witness in his own right to assess the high degree of intellectual, social and physiological recovery of somatic functions on the ipsilateral side of the body. While being observed during one year, his sensory recognition of objects and of weights steadily gained in accuracy, revealing that his remaining hemisphere was capable of utilizing ipsilateral data more fully as time progressed.

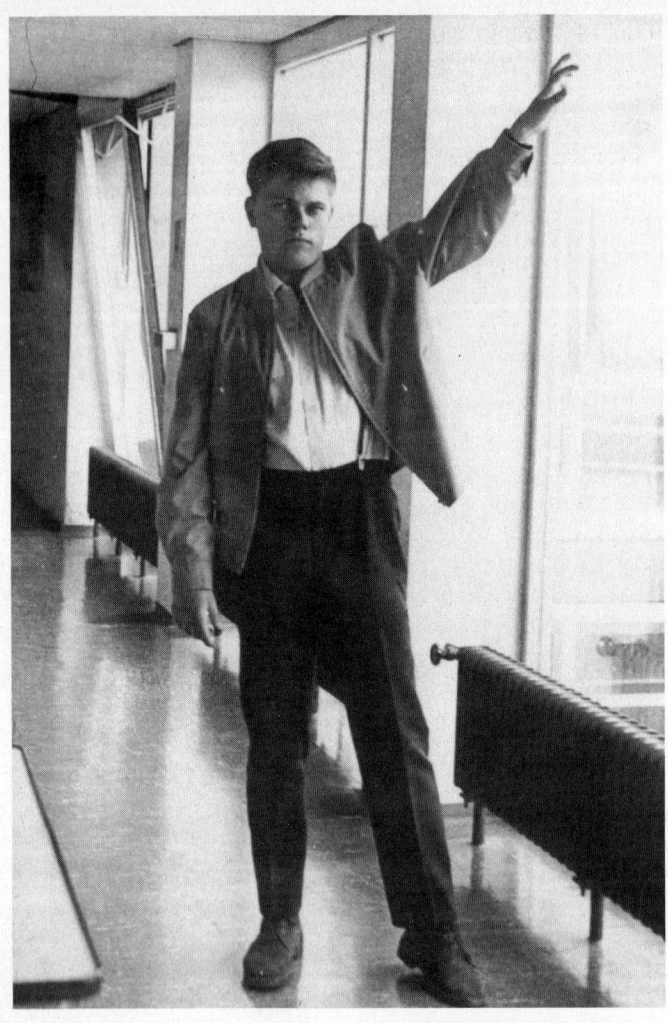

Figure 3. Patient of Dr. Boehnke, Hamburg, after right hemispherectomy, using his left spastic hand with fair skill.

Experimental investigations

To study preservations and retraining abilities of somatic functions after cortical lesions, experiments are reviewed which were performed in macaques and baboons having been trained previously for a number of dexterity and recognition tasks (GLEES, 1952, 1953, 1960, 1961; GLEES et al., 1950a, 1950b, 1951, 1952, 1958, 1973). Single, repeated and multiple lesions in the sensorimotor cortex were caused and the effects of these lesions and the time course studied.

The motor cortex

Electrical stimulation of the precentral gyrus or primary somatic motor area reveals repeatable somatotopic organization well known to all investigators of cortical motor function (reviewed by GLEES, 1961), e.g., in every primate subject studied by stimulation, the thumb area is sharply separated from the face area, and the boundary is outlined by a small artery. Taking the constant and reliable motor responses into account, one is not surprised that after ablation of the hand area, disability of hand skill is very evident. Our studies of sensorimotor skill were mainly concentrated on hand skill, using the problem box, the dexterity board, a shape-discriminating board and differently shaped objects hidden in a bag (Figures 4 and 5). These tests have been described by GLEES (1961).

As for the recovery of function after cortical lesions, the loss of the skillful use of the hand after lesions in the hand area is only temporary and is completely restored after a few weeks. If, then, another lesion is made in an area adjacent to that already destroyed, there is a renewed loss of function and renewed subsequent recovery of learned motor functions (LASHLEY, 1929). If the motor cortex were indeed a mosaic, then the destruction of one portion should produce a permanent loss of function. The question therefore is: What is responsible for the recovery of skilled motor function? The work of GRÜNBAUM & SHERRINGTON (1903), SHERRINGTON

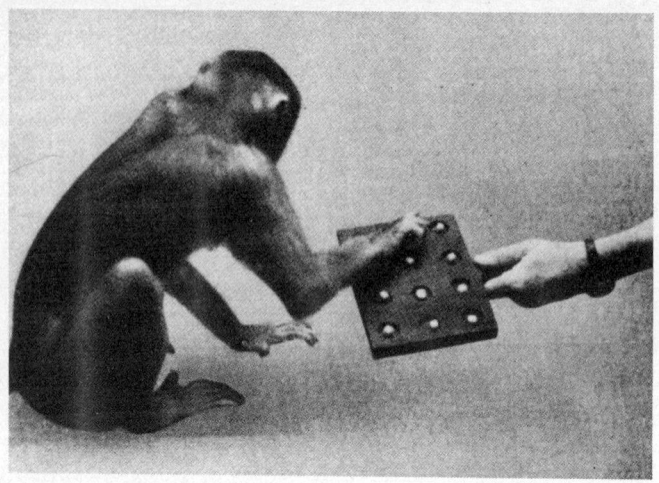

Figure 4. Right hand of a pigtail monkey carrying out a skilled task.

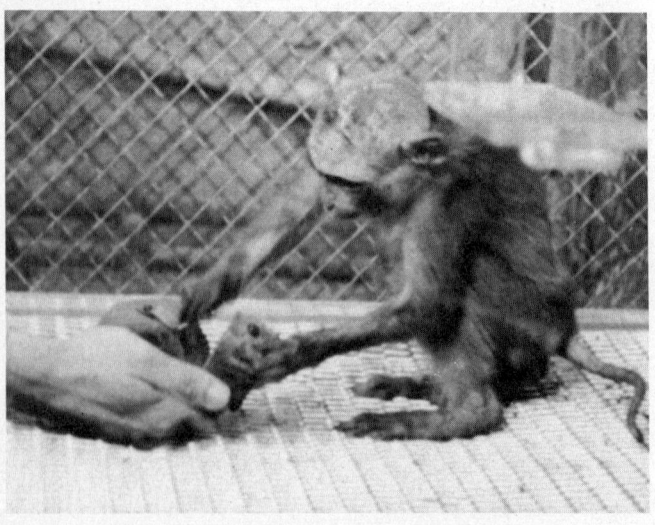

Figure 5. Recovery of right hand motor function after left motor cortex lesion. The monkey is again capable of opening the problem box.

(1906), SCHÜLLER (1906), and ROTHMANN (1907) on motor recovery was based on the idea that subcortical centers compensate for the loss of motor cortex. In this, however, the fact that motor function has several levels of organization was completely overlooked. As we have seen, primitive functions are controlled not by the cortex, but by the midbrain or forebrain. It is therefore not surprising that a monkey can still grab food and climb around its cage without a motor cortex, after the direct effects of the operation have subsided. To suppose that these primitive functions were cortical in origin was mistaken. Cortically controlled function must be studied in animals which can be trained before operation to perform certain actions requiring skill. Their performance after operation is measured and any loss of dexterity recorded. In this way, the effects of the removal of cortical areas are seen in the less primitive motor actions which are above subcortical control. The rhesus monkey and pigtail monkey, which are very docile, have proved very suitable animals to train for such experiments.

The sensory cortex

The initial effects of lesions made in the sensory cortex in monkeys involve loss of dexterity and the power to discriminate between different shapes. There is also a loss of tone in the arms. Some animals do not seem to be aware of the position of their arms and will hold them for a considerable time in unusual or uncomfortable positions.

There is, however, a considerable degree of recovery from these disabilities, which can be measured by using monkeys trained before operation and again tested on their performance postoperatively.

Discussion

Limiting factors for rehabilitation or functional reorganization after hemispherectomy are the degree and duration of epilepsy in conjunction with the type of relevant treatment, the basic pretraumatic personality and its genetics and the postoperative care and schooling or retraining given (cf., Munz & Tolor, 1955).

One important factor is valid for all cases: the bilaterality of one hemisphere as far as motor performance and sensory recognition is concerned. Even where the diseased and eventually removed hemisphere resulted in reduced motor control (cf., case 2), this initial loss can be recovered by the ipsilateral fiber component of the remaining hemisphere (Figures 6–11).

Unfortunately, the full usage of the ipsilateral pyramidal fibers is very much reduced as far as the hand is concerned, as spasticity in flexion is very much in the foreground. If the fingers are brought passively in extension, voluntary flexion of thumb and index finger can be executed well by the patient. For fuller rehabilitation, it would be vital to be able to reduce or abolish the spastic interference. But in any case, it is comforting for accident or stroke patients to realize that one hemisphere, on account of ipsilateral fibers, has the potentiality

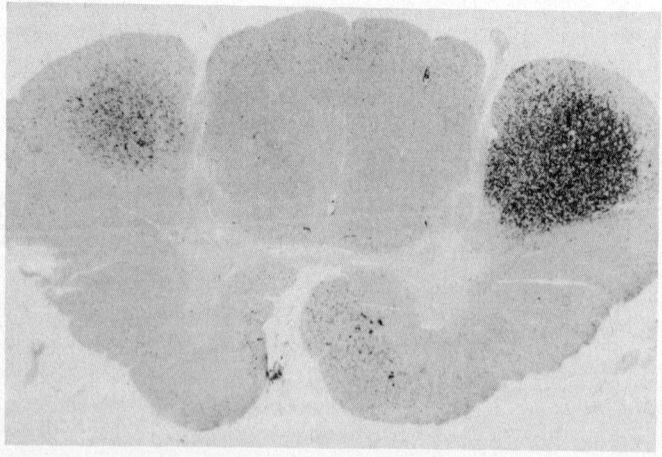

Figure 6. Degeneration of spinal pyramidal fibers in man shown in a late Marchi stage, one year after injury to one hemisphere. It shows the large area of crossed and uncrossed ipsilateral pyramidal fibers at the C6 level. This case illustrates that man has a fair amount of uncrossed fibers intermingling with those of the crossed tract.

to produce limited motor power in a spastic limb and all therapeutic effects should be directed towards this aim; namely, to retrain ipsilateral motor power, even in patients older than the cases reported here.

One of the patients (PG) (the most intelligent and cooperative among the 18 patients) had his right hemisphere removed by the late Sir HUGH CAIRNS on March 14, 1950, and subsequently was extensively studied. In sensory testing of his left side over a period of months he showed a considerable improvement in sensory recognition of shapes and cutaneous location of pain and fine touch. PG was also one of the patients included in a followup study by GRIFFITH & DAVIDSON (1966) over a period of 15 years. They reported that this patient had obtained a university diploma and held a responsible administrative position with a local authority. This patient proved convincingly that one hemisphere is sufficient as a substratum for an apparently complete personality. The pa-

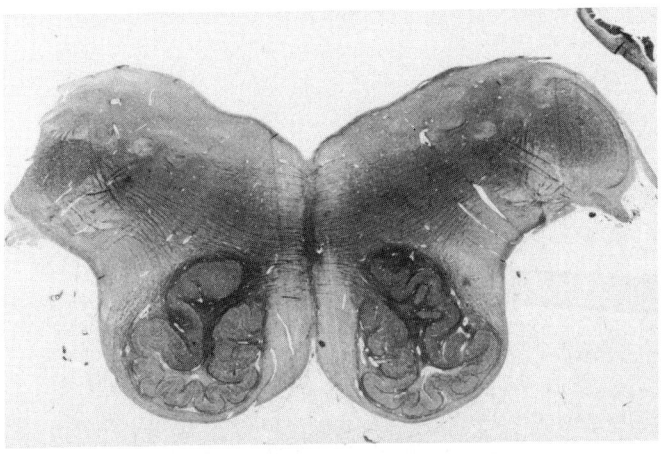

Figure 7. The size of the pyramidal tract area is a safe and clear indication of whether the impairment occurred during pregnancy, in infancy or in later life from a cerebral trauma. The medulla of a hydrocephalic patient who survived several months after birth: due to the expanding hydrocephalic cerebral hemisphere, the descending pyramidal fibers were unable to reach the medullary level of the brainstem and a pyramidal tract is missing on both sides.

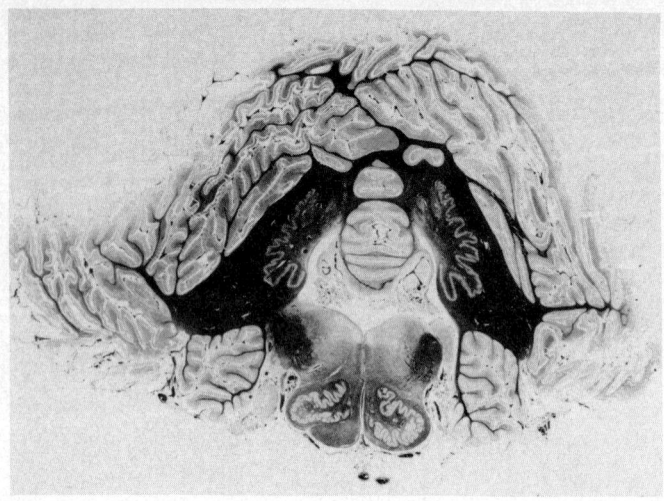

Figure 8. A case of infantile spastic hemiplegia. Note the absence of one pyramid.

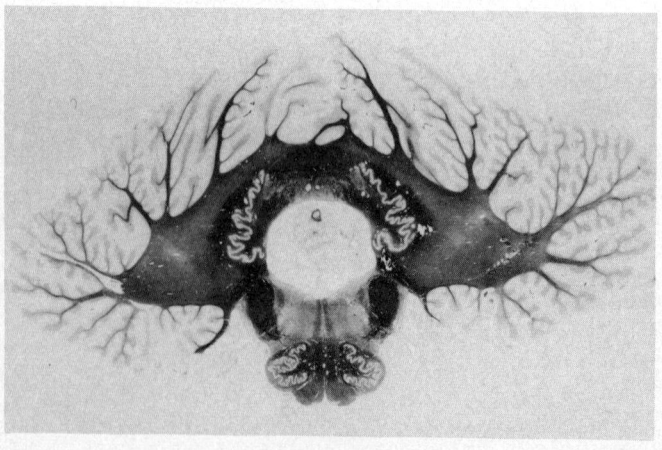

Figure 9. Normal human medulla to show the equal size of both pyramidal areas.

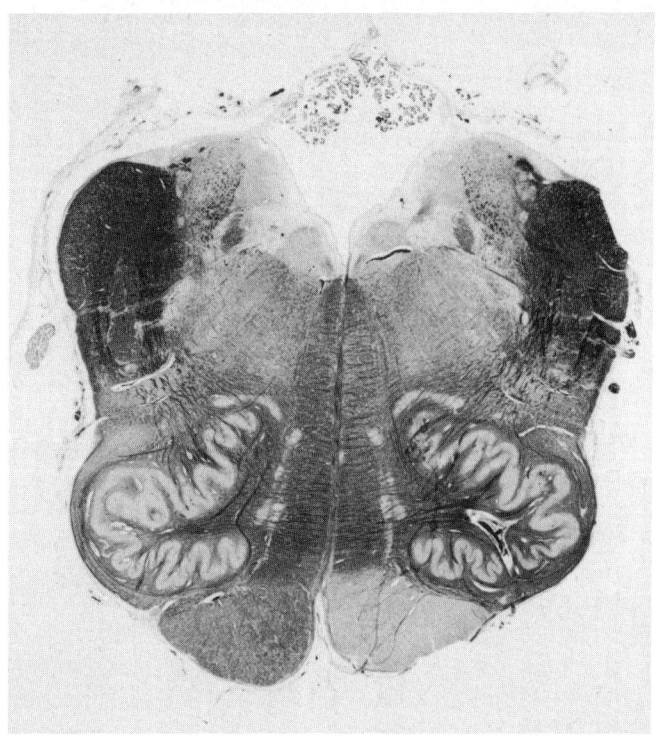

Figure 10. Following brain injury to one hemisphere, the postmortem study (one year after accident) reveals an absence of all pyramidal fibers on one side, but the pyramidal area, as such, has preserved its original size.

tients not only control the opposite half of the body, but have the ipsilateral half of the body integrated into the mental events of the surviving hemisphere. Obviously the motor control of the ipsilateral half of the body is reduced for two reasons: the ipsilateral corticospinal component of the surviving hemisphere is insufficient in numbers, especially concerning the hand muscles, and the spasticity prevents full rehabilitation. Concerning the corticopontine and corticospinal pathway from the remaining hemisphere, the impression prevails that these pathways are more numerous and the average fibers more thickly myelinated than in normal brain tissue.

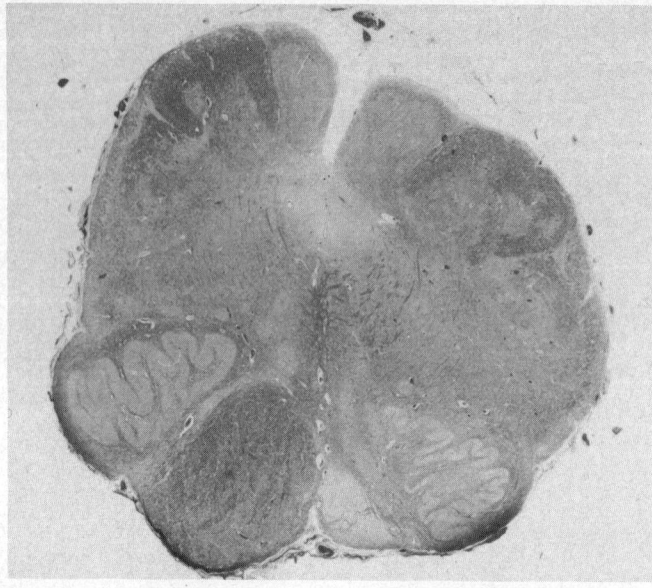

Figure 11. The medulla at the level of the nuclei of Goll and Burdach. Note the great reduction of one pyramidal area. The remaining pyramidal area is grossly reduced in size due to the degeneration of pyramidal fibers in early infancy. However, at close inspection, this pyramidal area is divided in two different atrophic portions. The ventral one is the residual area caused by the early degeneration, the dorsal and lighter area was filled by surviving pyramidal fibers now degenerated by the removal of the ipsilateral hemisphere.

Experimental findings support this view and Sammeck (1976, 1977, 1978) found in rats that use or disuse of the motor system has a direct effect on motor fiber size and myelin thickness.

It is therefore of great importance for rehabilitation training programs to exercise all pathways from the deprived half of the body to the preserved hemisphere and vice versa.

Noteworthy too is the preservation of speech. It is certain that the speech areas will move to the undamaged hemisphere in cases of infantile hemiplegia and that this sole hemisphere can draw upon its own large reservoir, having no minor hemisphere for reference, in contrast to the commisurral observations by Butler & Norrsell (1968). In this connection, reference must be made to the discussion of GRIFFITH's & DAVIDSON's paper on long term changes in intellect and behavior (1966) when referring to the aspects of cerebral dominance and whether a patient would be better off with a left or right hemisphere lesion. This view is based on the assumption that the nondominant hemisphere has spatial and constructional functions. The authors believe that less intelligent patients aiming at practical, nonverbal skills would be better off with a left hemisphere lesion, while an intelligent hemiplegic would seem to be better off with a left hemiplegia, as the acquisition of verbal skills could compensate for his physical handicaps by the intact left hemisphere.

Concerning the surgical removal of one hemisphere (e.g., the left in DW), I was struck that the histological examination of the prefrontal cortex, the sensorimotor cortex and the temporal lobe revealed no abnormalities. Physiologically, some part of the left motor cortex were functioning, since at operation, electrical stimulation gave motor responses in the right arm, and after operation, a transient weakness was observable in the right arm. The corpus callosum appeared normal too, but the removal of the left hemisphere was without significant effect on verbal and sensorimotor behavior. In this case, all main cerebral activities were assembled in the right hemisphere, leaving an anatomically preserved left hemisphere apparently unused. It is surprising too that the removal of one hemisphere does not lead to disturbance of consciousness or at least a reduction in the level of consciousness. This is not even noticeable immediately after recovery from operation. Consciousness cannot therefore rely on interhemispheric connections or by being able to mirror mental events in the opposite hemisphere. CHAPMAN & WOLFF (1959), in their excellent review on cerebral function, state, «... that considerable portions of one or both hemispheres can be removed without complete loss of consciousness, and when one hemisphere is badly damaged in infancy, it can be removed in later life without additional impairment. From our cases it can be concluded that an efficient level of consciousness can be maintained by one hemisphere and its subcortical connections.» However, another case (RL), reported by OPPENHEI-

MER & GRIFFITH (1966), showed a severe destruction in the hemisphere removed, and during life, exhibited a very much reduced personality (GLEES & WHITE, unpublished). It seems then that an intact callosal system can transfer information continuously to the leading hemisphere until surgical intervention terminates this possibility. Unfortunately, corpus callosum function has been discussed very little in papers on hemispherectomy, nor has attention been paid to the fact that massive callosal system degeneration must occur as the result of one hemisphere removal, with both terminal degeneration of stem fibers from the removed side, and cell soma changes due to its fiber severance by hemispherectomy. It seems that the subsequent cell loss of the callosal distribution system has no significant effects on postoperative intelligence; GRIFFITH & DAVIDSON (1966) remark that 5 out of 12 patients have made worthwhile progress in intelligence over the years observed. This could mean that the callosal system only carries information, but plays no role in preservation or elaboration of information. This view is supported by the primate experiments of EBNER & MYERS (1962) who found no depression of learning through the separate body members in monkeys after section of the corpus callosum, while crossrecognition between the hands or feet for tactile learning was abolished. Total hemispherectomy in the monkey performed by WHITE et al. (1959) showed that bilateral motor function is excellent and supports the view that each hemisphere has a bilateral cortical outflow. The paper presented by WHITE et al. (1959) should also be consulted for its review of the relevant experimental data.

From the study of the course of degenerating cortical fibers after small lesions, it is concluded that, though a particular subdivision (e.g., the hand area) of the motor cortex sends most of its descending fibers to the appropriate segments of the cervical cord, a minority of fibers are connected with other levels as well. This could be proved for all subdivisions of area 4. These plurisegmental connections of the major subdivisions of the motor cortex within the cord offer an explanation of motor recovery subsequent to small lesions in area 4. The concept of plurisegmental connections from the cortex most readily explains functional recovery and would do more justice to the embryological descent of corticofugal fibers, which appear to connect with all spinal levels, to start with and achieve a more selected mode of projection during maturation.

Electrical cortical stimulation of cortical regions close to the small lesions give motor responses previously only obtainable from the now ablated area. As long as a portion of the primary motor cortex is preserved, contralateral movement patterns can be elicited.

Recovery of sensory function after lesion in the primary sensory cortex

Motor power returns to normal, although dexterity remains permanently affected, but the most striking recovery is the complete return of stereognosis. Even after ablation of the hand region, the monkey is able to differentiate by touch between a cone and a pyramid, after only a few weeks (COLE & GLEES, 1953). This confirms the findings of RUCH (1935) that a monkey (cerocebus torquatos atys) trained to discriminate between different weights was still able to do so after ablation of the sensory cortical region.

If the sensory impulses from the periphery were projected solely through selected regions of the thalamus and sensory cortex, no such recovery of function would be possible.

There must therefore be additional pathways which, by facilitation, affected by postoperative training, are brought into direct sensory contact with other intact portions of the cortex. After the ablation of the hand region of the sensory cortex, the peripheral impulses from the hand may be transmitted from the hand region of the thalamus to another, intact part of the sensory cortex, or there may be alternative pathways which take impulses from the hand to regions of the thalamus other than the hand region, whence the normal pathway to the appropriate region of the sensory cortex takes over. Other reserve pathways must then also exist to enable the sensory signals to reach the motor cortex by an alternative route (GLEES, 1953). It is also possible that the motor cortex receives sensory information from the thalamus via the superior cerebellar peduncle (WEINSTEIN et al., 1940). Since the alternative route will normally be little used, postoperative training is of the utmost importance. The operated animal will refuse to use its damaged arm unless there is some incentive to do so, and its cooperation must be gained by attractive food reward enticement. If these observations are applied to clinical neurology, it is most likely that persistent physiotherapy may be the means of producing a certain degree of functional recovery and rehabilitation after cortical injury. No doubt the patient should be more willing to cooperate than some operated monkeys.

Summary

The degree of rehabilitation and functional recovery is assessed in human cases of hemispherectomy and in experiments in primates following small lesions in the sensorimotor cortex.

1) Motivation and postoperative care are essential factors for the return of function in both motor and sensory disabled limbs.
2) In particular, the management of the whole body by one hemisphere alone is a surprising fact, morphologically supported by the presence and utilization of unused or rerouted pathways and of ipsilateral connections for motor and sensory pathways.
3) Corpus callosum function needs further exploration in view of the fact that this system has been destroyed by hemispherectomy, without causing definite deficits.

Acknowledgements

My thanks are due to Mr. J. F. Crane and R. Dungan for the illustrations and to Mrs. F. Glees for the preparation of the manuscript.

Bibliography

Addendum: In the framework of my contribution I would like to draw attention to two valuable clinical papers a) BRODAL, A.: Self-observations and neuro-anatomical considerations after a stroke, Brain *96,* 675–694, 1973, which is extremely relevant to rehabilitation problems.

b) JUNG, R., DIETZ, V.: Verzögerter Start der Willkürbewegung bei Pyramidenläsionen des Menschen. Arch.Psychiat.Nervenkr. *221,* 87–109, 1975, where the authors emphasize the functional importance of homolateral or uncrossed pyramidal fibres.

BUTLER, S.R., NORRSELL, U.: Vocalization possibly initiated by the minor hemisphere. Nature *220,* 793, Nov.23, 1968.

CHAPMAN, L.F., WOLFF, H.G.: The cerebral hemispheres and the highest integrative functions of man. A.M.A. Arch.Neurol. *1,* 357, Oct.1959.

EBNER, F.F., MYERS, R.E.: Corpus callosum and the interhemispheric transmission of tactual learning. J.Neurophysiol. *25,* 380, 1962.

FABISCH, W., GLEES, P., McMILLAN, A.L.: Hemispherectomy for the treatment of epilepsy in infantile hemiplegia. Mschr.Psychiat.Neurol. *130,* 6, 1955.

GLEES, P.: Leistungsfähigkeit von Menschen mit nur einer Hirnhälfte. Umschau, Heft 14, 64–65, 1952.

GLEES, P.: The interrelation of the thalamus and the sensorimotor cortex. Mschr. Psychiat.Neurol. *125,* 129, 1953.

GLEES, P.: Analyse von Faktoren, welche die Darstellung der Terminal degeneration beeinflussen, mit einem Hinweis auf die Pyramidenbahn. Verh.Anat. Ges. (Jena) *187,* 56, 1959.

GLEES, P.: Experimental Neurology. Oxford: Clarendon Press, 1961, pp.532.

GLEES, P.: Contra- and ipsilateral motor and sensory representation in the cerebral cortex of monkey. In: Zülch, K.J., Creutzfeldt, O., Galbraith, G.C. (Eds): Cerebral Localization. Springer, Berlin/Heidelberg/ New York, 1975, pp.48.

GLEES, P., COLE, J., LIDDELL, E.G.T., PHILLIPS, C.G.: Beobachtungen über die motorische Rinde des Affen. Arch.Psychiat.Z.Neurol. *185,* 675, 1950.

GLEES, P., COLE, J.: Recovery of skilled motor functions after small repeated lesions in motor cortex in macaque. J.Neurophysiol. *13,* 137, 1950a.

GLEES, P., COLE, J.: Beobachtungen über Wiederherstellung der motorischen Funktionen nach Rindenabtragung beim Rhesusaffen. Verh.d. Dtsch.Zool. Mainz *1949,* 198–201, 1950b.

GLEES, P., WHITE, W.G.: Resettlement of a case of hemispherectomy for the treatment of infantile hemiplegia. Trans.Ass.Industr.Med.Officers *7,* 127, 1958.

GLEES, P., NOVOTNY, G.E.K., SPOERRI, O.: Pyramidenbahn und primäre motorische Rinde, Neurobiologie, Klinische Demonstration. Institut f.d. Wissenschaftlichen Film, Wissenschaftlicher Film C 1122/1973, Göttingen (W.Germany), 1974.

GRIFFITH, H., DAVIDSON, M.: Long-term changes in intellect and behavior after hemispherectomy. J.Neurol.Neurosurg.Psychiat. *29,* 571, 1966.

GRÜNBAUM, R.S.F., SHERRINGTON, C.S.: Observations on the physiology of the cerebral cortex of the anthropoid apes. Proc.Roy.Soc. *72,* 152, 1903.

LASHLEY, K.S.: Brain Mechanisms and Intelligence. N.Y.: Dover Publ., 1963, pp.186.

MUNZ, A., TOLOR, A.: Psychological affects of major cerebral excision: Intellectual and emotional changes following hemispherectomy. J.Nerv. Ment.Dis. *121,* 438, 1955.

OPPENHEIMER, D.R., GRIFFITH, H.B.: Persistent intracranial bleeding as a complication of hemispherectomy. J.Neurol.Neurosurg.Psychiat. *29,* 229, 1966.

ROTHMANN, N.: Über die physiologische Wertung der cortico-spinalen (Pyramiden-)Bahn. Arch.Anat.Physiol. *31,* 217, 1907.

RUCH, T.C.: Cortical localization of somatic sensibility. The effect of precentral, postcentral and posterior parietal lesions upon the performance of monkeys trained to discriminate weights. Res.Publ.Ass.Nerv.Ment. Dis. *15,* 289, 1935.

SAMMECK, R.: Myelin changes induced by detraining. Proceedings of the Physiological Society, Dec. 1976, J.Physiol. *266,* 16, 1976.

SAMMECK, R.: An experimental model to induce myelination in adult animals. Proc. Internat.Soc.Neurochem. *6,* 585, 1977.

SAMMECK, R.: Studying myelination as a parameter of function. Trans.Amer.Soc. Neurochem. *9,* 176, 1978.

SCHÜLLER, A.: Experimentelle Pyramidendurchschneidung beim Hunde und Affen. Wien.klin.Wschr. *19,* 57, 1906.

SHERRINGTON, C.S.: The Integrative Action of the Nervous System. N.Y., C.Scrib. Sons, 1906, pp.411.

WEINSTEIN, E., SJOQVIST, O., FULTON, J.F.: Effect of medial lemniscus section on weight discrimination. Amer.J.Physiol. *129,* 491, 1940.

WHITE, R.J., SCHREINER, L.H., HUGHES, R.A., MAC CARTY, C.S., GRINDLAY, J.H.: Physiologic consequences of total hemispherectomy in the monkey. Neurology, 1958, *9,* 3, 1959.

Animal models for effects of brain lesions and for rehabilitation

MARK R. ROSENZWEIG

I. Introduction

While four of the papers in this symposium are devoted mainly or entirely to studies of human subjects, three are based in large part on research with animal subjects. The present chapter examines ways in which the two sorts of studies are related – how work with animal models has contributed and may contribute further to rehabilitation of human patients and also how studies of human patients have and can contribute toward greater understanding of brain-behavior relations in animals. Not only contributions but also problems of extrapolation and interpretation and limitations of cross-species comparisons will be considered.

Models are widely used in scientific research, and animal models are frequently employed to study both disease processes and also normal behavior in human beings. Often the value of such models is accepted implicitly, but several investigators have recently shown explicit concern with development of animal models (e.g., BEACH, in press; HANIN & USDIN, Eds., 1977; HARLOW et al., 1972; LIPTON et al., 1978, pp.553–620; MORRISON & MCKINNEY, 1976; WARREN & KOLB, 1978). The majority of the chapters in several recent books on recovery of function are based on research with animal subjects (FINGER, 1978a; STEIN, ROSEN & BUTTERS, 1974; WALSH & GREENOUGH, 1976). In this paper I will review some selected examples, considering the possible relevance of such models for developments in rehabilitation. Two sets of examples will be given. In the first set, much of the research was specifically intended to deal with possible methods of rehabilitation. In the second set, the main impetus for research was the attempt to resolve apparent discrepancies between human beings and other animals in certain brain-behavior relationships; some of the results of this research also have implications for rehabilitation. In the last section of the chapter, I will examine some generalizations about the use of animal models in this field of research.

II. Animal models for effects of brain lesions and for rehabilitation

The psychologist SHEPARD IVORY FRANZ (1874–1933) was a pioneer in the use of animal models to study cerebral mechanisms of behavior and in attempts to apply the results to rehabilitation. At the start of this century he was the first to combine the method of localized ablation with the new methods of studying animal learning that had recently been described by THORNDIKE in 1898. FRANZ (1902) hoped to localize regions of the brain that were specifically responsible for learning and memory, but he concluded on the basis of his experimental results that these properties are not localized in any region of the brain but, on the contrary, are widely dispersed. When KARL S. LASHLEY was a graduate student, he collaborated with FRANZ on further experiments of this sort, and out of this research developed the program of LASHLEY's long career. During and after the first World War, FRANZ attempted to employ psychological methods of training and motivation to rehabilitate injured soldiers, and LASHLEY also participated in some of this work. It was a major regret of FRANZ that he was not able to persuade federal authorities to initiate a massive program of research and application in rehabilitation (FRANZ, 1932; WOODWORTH, 1934).

Continuing from the research initiated by FRANZ and carried on by LASHLEY, many investigators have used animal subjects to study how brain lesions affect learning and memory, and also the extent to which various programs of experience and/or training can overcome or minimize effects of brain lesions. A recent chapter (GREENOUGH, FASS & DEVOOGD, 1976) has reviewed the influence of experience on recovery of function depending upon whether the experience was provided (a) prior to the lesion, (b) between two successive lesions separated by weeks or months, or (c) following the lesion. I will discuss research on the latter two points and will also take up the possibilities of secondary and continued cerebral degeneration after a circumscribed lesion, behavioral implications of such degeneration, and possible effects of experience upon it.

A. Effects of postlesion experience on recovery of function

A major question concerning recovery of function following brain injury is this: Which of the following types of treatment is best suited to promote the highest possible level of recovery? (a) Working simply to restore general health, on the assumption that this will automatically aid the fullest possible restoration of function. (b) Giving special experience and/or training tailored to the functional deficits shown by the individual. (c) Protecting the individual from stimulation so that the impaired nervous system is not overloaded. Each of these types of therapy has been espoused and put into practice by different clinicians, but direct comparisons between the results have rarely been made. This is the kind of situation in which well-designed experiments with human patients are difficult to initiate and carry out, but where research on animal models is quite feasible.

A more fundamental question concerns the neural mechanism(s) involved in recovery of function. Several hypotheses have been proposed, each appearing to account for certain clinical observations. If it could be determined which hypothesis is correct, or under what conditions different hypotheses are correct, this would have important consequences for designing effective programs of rehabilitation. Again, research with animal models allows more direct experimentation with neural mechanisms than does clinical observation or experiments with human subjects.

Rather than review effects of enriching or restricting experience on recovery of a broad range of behaviors including motivational and emotional behavior, as did GREENOUGH et al. (1976), we will concentrate on studies of maze-learning ability. Removal of small amounts of cerebral cortex has long been known to impair learning scores in laboratory animals. In a widely-cited single experiment, SCHWARTZ (1964) demonstrated that allowing rats to experience an enriched environment for three months postlesion significantly improved their test scores. SCHWARTZ made lesions in occipital cortex of some rat pups on the day after birth and made sham operations in others. He assigned the pups after weaning either to the usual colony cages or to a more enriched condition (EC). EC consisted in a large cage housing a dozen animals and containing varied stimulus objects. At about 120 days of age the rats were pretrained and then tested in the standard series of 12 problems in the Hebb-Williams maze. Scores of rats from the four experimental conditions are shown in Table 1. Brain-lesioned rats from the enriched environment scored as well as did rats with intact brains from the colony environment; best of all were rats with intact brains and enriched experience, and worst were rats with lesions and restricted experience.

Our research group decided to attempt to replicate and extend this interesting experiment for several reasons: (a) We had found in an extensive program of research that we could induce significant changes in brain anatomy and brain chemistry by giving rats differential experience in one of three environments – standard colony cages (SC), a more enriched condition (EC), or isolated in an impoverished condition (IC) (BENNETT et al., 1964; BENNETT, 1976; ROSENZWEIG & BENNETT, 1976, 1977, 1978). These effects of differential experience on brain measures will be reviewed briefly in the next

Table 1. Mean errors on Hebb-Williams maze as function of neonatal cortical lesions and postlesion environment. (Values from Fig.1, SCHWARTZ, 1964.)

Postoperative environment	Brain status	
	Lesioned	Intact
Standard colony	205	125
Enriched	95	65

paragraphs. Since experience has measurable effects on the brain, it seemed worthwhile to test whether behavioral recovery after the lesion might be related to the cerebral effects of enriched experience. (b) We had found that these cerebral effects of experience could be enhanced by giving rats small doses of excitant drugs in the enriched environment (BENNETT et al., 1973; ROSENZWEIG & BENNETT, 1972). Since excitant drugs have been reported to promote recovery after brain lesions (e.g., WARD & KENNARD, 1942; MEYER et al., 1963), we suggested that a combination of enriched experience and an excitant drug might be particularly effective in aiding recovery (BENNETT et al., 1973). (c) SCHWARTZ's experiment included only neonatal operations, and it seemed important to determine whether experience could also help to overcome effects of lesions inflicted later in life. (d) Finally, the enriched condition includes a number of aspects, with both social and inanimate stimulation, and we wanted to determine whether certain aspects of EC are more important than others in promoting recovery of maze-solving ability.

1. Effects of experience on brain in intact animals

Cerebral effects of experience in enriched (EC), standard colony (SC), or impoverished (IC) environments were first sought in experiments done to follow up an unexpected observation: Groups of rats that had been made to solve tasks varying in difficulty were found to differ in activity of the enzyme acetylcholinesterase (AChE) in the cerebral cortex (ROSENZWEIG, KRECH & BENNETT, 1961). The differential environments were then used to provide the opportunity for widely differing amounts of self-paced learning. The enriched condition (EC) used in our laboratory consisted in housing a group of 10–12 same-sex rats in a large cage ($76 \times 76 \times 45$ cm) and placing about 6 stimulus objects in the cage each day from a pool of about 25 objects (wooden bar, metal box, lightbulb, pan with wood shavings, etc.). Stimulus objects that we commonly use are shown in Figure 2 of ROSENZWEIG and BENNETT (1969). In the standard colony condition (SC), three rats were caged together in a small colony cage ($21 \times 34 \times$

20 cm); any cage that meets standards for animal cage is adequate for this purpose. For the impoverished condition (IC), animals were housed individually in colony cages. In our early work, the IC subjects were housed in cages with solid side walls (as shown in the drawing of all three conditions in ROSENZWEIG et al., 1972a, p. 23), and the IC cages were placed in quiet and dimly illuminated rooms. We later found that extracage stimulation is of little importance for rats, so in many experiments we have housed IC and SC rats in the same kind of cage and on the same racks.

Exposure to the EC, SC, or IC environments from 25 to 105 days of age was found to produce significant differences, not only in cortical AChE but also in weight of standard samples of the cortex (ROSENZWEIG et al., 1962). These changes did not represent simply a general growth of the brain because they were considerably larger in the cortex than in the rest of the brain, and within the cortex they were largest in the occipital area where the difference in weight between EC and IC littermates often amounts to about 10%. Further regional specificity will be seen when we examine effects of differential experience on the anatomy of cortical neurons.

Table 2 presents representative brain weight values for rats from the SC condition, and it also gives percentage differences for EC versus SC, IC versus SC, and EC versus IC rats. These values are based on littermate rats assigned at random to the three conditions at weaning (25 days of age) and kept there for 30 days. Data from similar experiments lasting from 25 to 105 days of age are given in ROSENZWEIG et al., (1972, Table 3). Note in Table 2 that there was a significant difference between EC and IC rats in each of the areas of the cortex that was studied, with the largest difference in the occipital area; there was not a significant difference in the rest of the brain (subcortex). A particularly stable measure of differential experience is the ratio of weight of total cortex to weight of the rest of the brain (cortical/subcortical ratio). This ratio yields, in effect, a value adjusted for covariance of brain weights on body weights (ROSENZWEIG et al., 1972b, pp. 229–230, 236–237). It should be emphasized that the differences in brain weight between EC and IC rats cannot be attributed to

Table 2. Differences among EC, SC, and IC rats in brain weights (mg) and body weights (gm)[1].

	SC Mean ± standard deviation	EC versus SC		IC versus SC		EC versus IC	
		% Diff.[2]	Number EC > SC[3]	% Diff.	Number IC > SC	% Diff.	Number EC > IC
Cortex							
Occipital	66 ± 4	3.3***	58	-5.6***	25	9.4***	71
Somesthetic	56 ± 4	-0.9	41.5	-4.3***	24	3.6***	64
Remaining dorsal	290 ± 16	1.0	48.5	-2.6***	26	3.7***	61
Ventral	246 ± 16	1.5	48	-1.9*	38	3.4***	58
Total	658 ± 28	1.2**	52	-2.8***	19	4.2***	72
Rest of brain	833 ± 39	-0.5	43.5	0.5	47	- 0.9	35
Total brain	1491 ± 65	0.3	47	-1.0*	30	1.3**	56
Cortex Rest	.790 ± .020	1.7***	60	-3.3***	8	5.1***	82
Terminal body weight	181 ± 18	-6.1***	25	5.6***	54	-11.0***	20

[1] Based on 87 littermate sets of male rats of the Berkeley S_1 stock placed in differential conditions from 25 to 55 days of age.

[2] Percent difference between EC and SC means.

[3] The number of the 87 littermate pairs in which the EC value exceeded the SC value.

$* p > .05$, $** p > .01$, $*** p > .001$. Based on Duncan's New Multiple Range Test.

body weight differences; in fact, the brain weights of rats reared in EC environments regularly exceed those of animals reared in IC environments, whereas IC animals achieve higher terminal body weights than do EC animals.

The differences between EC and IC rats in weights of cortical samples probably reflect mainly differences in thickness of the cortex (DIAMOND, KRECH & ROSENZWEIG, 1964; ROSENZWEIG, BENNETT & DIAMOND, 1972b; WALSH et al., 1969). In thickness as in weight, the differences are larger in the occipital area than in other cortical regions.

The anatomical effects of differential experience have been studied further at both the light- and electron-microscopic levels, as reviewed in detail by ROSENZWEIG and BENNETT (1978). Most of these effects have been studied only in the occipital cortex, since this is the region that showed the largest changes in cortical weight, depth, and chemistry. The cell bodies and nuclei of cortical neurons are significantly larger in cross-section in EC than in IC littermates (DIAMOND et al., 1976). Dendrites show significantly more higher-order branches in EC than in IC rats; SC animals have intermediate values but are closer to IC than to EC littermates in higher-order branching (GREENOUGH, 1976). Basal dendrites are longer in EC than in SC rats; this difference is localized quite specifically since it occurs chiefly in the terminal segment of the dendrites rather than in the initial or intermediate segments (UYLINGS, KUYPERS & VELTMAN, 1978). EC rats have greater numbers of dendritic spines per unit length of dendrite than do IC littermates, and this effect is also localized within the neuron; it is largest for basal dendrites (9.7%, $p <$ .01), present for oblique dendrites (3.6%, $p < .05$), and absent for apical dendrites (GLOBUS et al., 1973). The size of synaptic contacts has been measured by electron microscopy in terms of the length of the postsynaptic opaque region in type I synapses in occipital cortex. Greater length of synaptic junctions in EC rats than in IC littermates has been reported by several groups (MØLLGAARD et al., 1971; WEST & GREENOUGH, 1972; DIAMOND et al., 1975; WALSH & CUMMINS, 1976). In related work, ALTSCHULER (1976) reported that 80 days of combined environmental enrichment and training led to a doubling of synaptic density in comparison with control rats.

The two cholinergic enzymes, acetylcholinesterase (AChE) and cholinesterase (ChE), were found to differ not only in the direction but also in the rate of response to EC versus IC experience. EC rats developed significantly less AChE activity per unit of cortical tissue weight than IC littermates, but the EC rats showed significantly greater ChE per unit of weight. While the differences in AChE were significant by 30 days in the experimental conditions, differences in ChE were often not apparent unless the experiment lasted longer – 60 or 80 days. «Whereas in 1964 we supposed that all of the cerebral effects we measured might be reflecting only different aspects of the same syndrome of changes, it now appears that various measures follow their own time courses and may eventually be shown to represent independent types of change» (ROSEN-ZWEIG et al., 1972b). The finding of a clear increase in ChE with enriched experience led us to look at numbers of glial cells. It was found that the cortex of EC rats had significantly greater numbers of glial cells than did that of IC littermates (DIAMOND et al., 1966).

Experiments in the 1960s indicated differences in nucleic acids in the cortex of EC and IC rats (ROSENZWEIG et al., 1972b), but we discontinued further work of this sort until the development of a more accurate and rapid method for analysis of RNA and DNA (MORIMOTO, FERCHMIN & BENNETT, 1974). The RNA/DNA ratio has since been found to be the most reliable chemical indicator of the EC-IC effect; in 90% of 550 pairs, the RNA/DNA ratio in the occipital cortex has

Table 3. Percentage differences in RNA, DNA, and weight of occipital cortex of 30 days of differential experience (EC versus IC) as a function of age at start.

Starting age (days)	27	102	202	303
No. of pairs	100	41	24	22
Tissue weight	8.4***	4.7**	2.7	3.6
RNA/DNA	9.6***	7.1***	9.4***	7.0***
RNA/weight	2.4***	1.4**	3.0***	1.7*
DNA/weight	-6.6***	-5.2***	-5.7***	-4.8***
Total RNA	11.0***	6.2***	5.7**	5.4*
Total DNA	1.3	-0.6	-3.4	1.3

been larger in the EC rat than in the IC littermate, and the average difference was 8% (ROSENZWEIG & BENNETT, 1978). Table 3 presents some comparisons between EC and IC littermates when rats spent 30 days in the differential environments, after having been placed in EC or IC at different starting ages. It will be seen that the RNA/DNA differences in occipital cortex of EC and IC rats were highly significant for all age groups. For values of RNA and DNA in the cortex of rats in various experiential conditions, see tables in ROSENZWEIG et al. (1978). The increased RNA in EC rats suggests heightened cerebral activity as a consequence of enriched experience.

Generality of EC-IC effects over strains and species. Significant EC-IC effects in weights of cortical samples and in either AChE and ChE in or RNA have been found in the several strains of laboratory rats tested to date – not only in the strains tested in our laboratories but also in the case of Sprague-Dawley rats (GELLER, 1971), Wistar rats (WALSH et al., 1971), and an albino line maintained in Argentina (FERCHMIN et al., 1970). The Berkeley strains were established in breeding colonies in the Netherlands in 1960, and the S_1 strain was recently investigated in regard to effects of EC and IC environments on cortical weights and AChE; typical effects were obtained (RAAIJMAKERS, 1978). Similar effects have also been obtained with other species of rodents – gerbils and inbred mice (ROSENZWEIG & BENNETT, 1969), feral deermice *(Peromyscus maniculatus)* (ROSENZWEIG & BENNETT, unpublished observations), and feral Belding's ground squirrels *(Speromophilus beldingi)* (ROSENZWEIG, SHERMAN & BENNETT, unpublished). Although such research has been confined to rodents until recently, work with monkeys is now beginning to be reported (FLOETER, GREENOUGH & SACKETT, 1978; GREENOUGH & JURASKA, in press).

Alternative interpretations of causes of EC-IC effects. Although the EC, SC, and IC environments were originally used in our research to provide opportunities for differential amounts of informal learning, we were concerned from the start with alternative interpretations of the cerebral effects. Thus we tested whether the effects could be attributed to differential locomotion or handling, and we found that this was

136

not the case. Subsequently we have tested and ruled out several other alternative interpretations, including stress, pituitary secretions, accelerated maturation, or social stimulation (Rosenzweig & Bennett, 1976, 1977). Recently we have shown that self-paced maze trials produce significant cerebral effects similar in distribution in the brain although smaller in magnitude than the EC effects (Bennett et al., in press). This, as well as evidence adduced by Greenough (1976), provides strong support for the position that the cerebral effects of differential experience are caused, at least in large part, by the neural processes involved in learning and storage of memory.

The picture that is emerging from these and related studies is that of a brain that is considerably more plastic than had been supposed in the 1940s and '50s (Rosenzweig & Bennett, in press). Even in the adult brain, measurable changes can be found as results of training or differential experience, and it is not necessary to employ harsh or extreme treatments such as stressors or sensory deprivation in order to produce such effects. Finding such plasticity in the adult brain raises questions about its possible relevance for learning and memory and also for recovery of function.

2. Effects of postlesion experience on recovery of function

In a series of experiments with rats of two strains, including both male and female subjects, we have found that enriched postlesion experience significantly aided subsequent performance in the Hebb-Williams maze. This was true not only when occipital cortex lesions were made in neonates (Will et al., 1976) but also postweaning (Will et al., 1977) and in young adults – rats over 100 days of age (Will & Rosenzweig, 1976). Although the enriched environment in most experiments was available 24 hours per day, a period of 2 hours per day was found to be as effective as 24 hours. The results with the maze test provide strong evidence that enriched experience promotes overall recovery of function: Good scores on the series of maze tests require a combination of sensorimotor capacities, motivation, learning and memory, and a deficit in any one of these capacities results in inferior performance. Comparable results of EC on recovery of function have also been obtained recently in an operant conditioning program involving auditory discrimination (WILL, 1978). Thus, at least for this animal model, there is now abundant evidence that optimal recovery is not obtained simply by restoration of general health, and certainly not by protecting the individual from stimulation as in the IC environment, but rather by providing complex stimulation and opportunities for experience.

Among the lesioned rats as among the sham-operated controls, the EC animals showed greater cortical weight and cortical RNA/DNA than the IC animals (WILL et al., 1977). This suggested that the improved behavioral recovery of the EC animals might have been mediated by (or at least directly related to) the observed cerebral effects of the enriched experience. Further research revealed, however, that this hypothesis was inadequate, as we shall see.

Use of methamphetamine in conjunction with the enriched condition did not produce better scores than a control saline solution in either lesioned or intact rats (WILL et al., 1977). In the publication of these results, we accounted for the lack of a predicted positive effect of the excitant drug in the following way: Behavioral observations showed that rats that received the drug in EC were more active than saline-injected controls for a few hours after the injection, but several hours later the drug-injected rats were less active; over a 24-hour period there was little difference in total activity. In a subsequent experiment, therefore, rats were placed in EC for only 2 hours per day and were given either methamphetamine or saline just before their daily period in EC. While EC had its usual beneficial effect, there was again no difference between drug and saline groups (WILL, SUTTER & OFFERLIN, 1977). This result was disappointing for two reasons. First, the attempt to augment the therapeutic effect was ineffective. Second, the behavioral effects were found not to be directly related to the measured cerebral effects, since the drug increased the cerebral measures but not the behavioral benefit; thus a simple hypothesis relating behavioral and cerebral effects of

138

enriched experience was infirmed, and other hypotheses must be developed and tested. The failure to find a drug effect in these experiments does not, of course, negate results obtained in other situations, as reviewed by BRAILOWSKY in this volume. It does, however, indicate that specific relations between deficit, drugs, and experience must be unraveled by patient research and that drug effects on recovery are not to be expected in every case.

In experiments recently completed, we have tested the effectiveness of social and inanimate stimuli in overcoming effects of cortical lesions on maze learning. Reasons for conducting these experiments were our findings that social stimulation could not completely account for the cerebral effects of various types of enriched experience (ROSENZWEIG et al., 1978), and that an enriched inanimate environment suffices to induce brain changes when rats are placed individually in EC, if they are primed to interact with the environment (ROSENZWEIG & BENNETT, 1972).

We have studied effects of the two kinds of postlesion enrichment on performance of rats in the Hebb-Williams series of maze patterns. Social enrichment was afforded by housing rats in a group of 12 in a large cage ($76 \times 76 \times 45$ cm) but not providing inanimate stimulus objects; we call this the Group Condition (GC). The enrichment afforded by experience with varied stimulus objects was added to social stimulation in the EC situation; here, as described earlier, the rats were not only housed in a group of 12 but they were given a new arrangement of stimulus objects each day. The impoverished-experience rats lived either singly in small colony cages in the first of the two experiments or three to a small colony cage in the second experiment. The earlier experiment (A in Fig.1) was run in 1977 and included 11 rats in each of the six experimental conditions. Experiment B, run in 1978, included 15 rats per group.

The behavioral results presented in Figure 1 show that both brain status (intact vs. lesioned) and postlesion environment determined the error scores. In each experiment the intact rats made significantly fewer errors than did those with brain lesions. Among the lesioned rats, those with postlesion

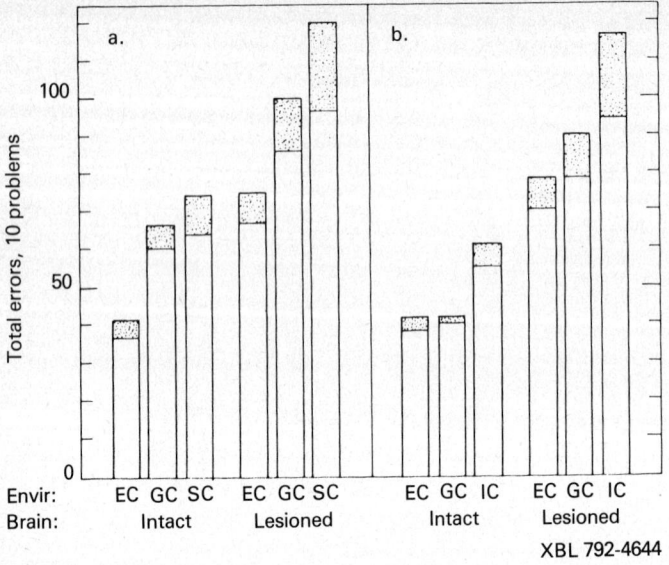

Figure 1. Error scores of rats, summed for ten problems of the Hebb-Williams maze. Postlesion environmental conditions were the following: EC, enriched condition with varied inanimate stimulus objects and social stimulation (rats housed 12 per large cage); GC, group condition, rats housed as in EC but without inanimate stimulus objects; SC, standard colony condition, rats housed 3 per small cage; IC, impoverished condition, rats housed singly in small colony cages. Height of bar shows total errors; these can be classified into initial errors (first error per trial in a given error zone, shown by the open portion of the bar) and repetitive errors (errors made after initial error, shown by stippled portion of the bar). Sections A and B of the figure report results of two successive experiments. See text for further description and for discussion of results.

experience enriched by the combination of inanimate and social experience (EC) made significantly fewer errors than did the impoverished-experience rats. In Experiment A, total errors of EC-lesioned rats were fewer than those of SC-lesioned rats at beyond the .01 level of confidence; in B, errors of EC-lesioned were less than those of IC-lesioned at beyond the .05 level. For the two experiments combined, the effect of this behavioral therapy was significant at beyond the .001 level of confidence. Social stimulation alone (GC) was less effective;

in neither experiment were the results of the GC-lesioned rats significantly different from those of the impoverished group (nor were they significantly different from those of the EC-lesioned group). For the two experiments combined, the errors of the GC-lesioned rats were fewer than those of the impoverished-experience rats (P < .05) but greater than those of EC-lesioned (P < .10). Thus the postoperative treatment (EC) that included inanimate as well as social stimulation was more effective than social stimulation alone (GC) in reducing the behavioral deficit caused by the cortical lesion.

Cortical lesions are not the only kinds of cerebral damage whose effects can be countered by enriched experience. Recently WILL et al. (in press) have demonstrated that the impairment in maze learning caused by hippocampal lesions can also be significantly diminished by experience in EC; the rats in this experiment were young adults (120 days of age) at the time the lesions were made. The learning deficits caused by inducing a hypothyroid condition in neonatal rats (experimental cretinism) have also been ameliorated by experience in enriched or «superenriched» environments (DAVENPORT, 1976). Infantile malnutrition in rodents does not invariably cause impairment in later learning – the literature is mixed in this regard (KATZ, 1977) – but one study has reported both clear impairment due to malnutrition and also significant remediation from enriched experience (WELLS, GEIST & ZIMMERMANN, 1972). Lead poisoning in rats impairs performance on a passive avoidance test; effects of a moderate dosage of lead were significantly remedied by enriched experience but those of a high dosage were not (PETIT & ALFANO, in press). Thus, enriched experience has been demonstrated to be beneficial in helping to overcome behavioral deficits that result from a variety of kinds of cerebral damage.

The question has been raised whether the improvement caused by enriched experience should properly be called recovery of function or whether it is simply an additive effect superimposed upon the effect caused by the lesion (PAUL R. CORNWELL, personal communication). This point was brought up in the discussion of an experiment in which cats were used as subjects; like the rats in the earlier experiments, the cats were subjected to either real or sham operations, and then they were housed in enriched or impoverished environments. The results for a cat-size Hebb-Williams maze were also similar, lesioned-EC cats performing significantly better than lesioned-IC cats and about as well as intact brain-IC animals. CORNWALL prefers to describe these results by stating simply that the lesions impair maze performance and enriched experience improves maze performance. As we have discussed previously (WILL et al., 1977), some experimental results do suggest interaction – greater effects of differential experience among lesioned than among intact subjects – but this is not invariably found nor is it necessarily valid because of problems of scales of measurement. What can be said at the least is that even damaged brains can benefit from experience and that their full capacity cannot be determined without training and/or enriched experience.

Results of these experiments demonstrate that, at least within this paradigm, the recovery of health does not guarantee the best possible recovery of problem-solving ability. Enriched experience helps, and not just any experience, since being in a social group had less effect than occurred when varied inanimate objects provided another kind of enrichment.

There is, of course, a growing body of research on effects of specific training in the rehabilitation of human patients. For example, BRUDNY et al. (1976) reported excellent results with feedback training to overcome disabling muscular activity; in many cases this therapy worked where other kinds had failed. MILLER (1978) has reviewed the use of biofeedback techniques for a variety of neurological disorders. While results have usually been favorable, there has been a lack of controlled studies that would be necessary to prove the value of these techniques. A highly successful program to retrain dysphasic patients has been reported from Australia (HOOPER, 1971). Several patients in this program actually found better jobs after training than they had held before their trauma. The report of the study stated that apparently these individuals had been «environmentally disadvantaged» (HOOPER, 1977, p.21) and that the clinic provided better opportunities for advancement than they had received before their accidents.

B. Lesion momentum – serial-lesion effects

It has long been recognized clinically that lesions that develop rapidly are more likely to produce symptoms than are those that develop slowly. Hughlings JACKSON in the last century wrote of symptomatology as related to «momentum of lesions» (mass times velocity). FINGER (1978b), in a recent review of this topic, stated that effects of lesion momentum on severity of symptoms have long been recognized. «Further, the rate of lesion development is one of a number of factors which can be invoked to account for intersubject variability on a wide range of neurological and behavioral tests designed to identify and localize brain damage. Nevertheless, in part because the principle is very difficult to assess under controlled conditions with human patient populations, it is discussed in minimal detail and is rarely referenced in most current textbooks and clinical monographs» (p. 137).

This may be the sort of situation in which research with animal models can help to make up for the lack of human data. It has been proposed that the lesion-momentum phenomenon can be studied through experiments with multiple successive lesions in animals; that is, experiments in which two or more small removals of tissue are spaced out over a period of days or weeks rather than all of the tissue being destroyed in a single operation. Many experiments comparing multiple-stage with single-stage lesions have been reported in recent years (see review by FINGER, 1978b).

Experimenters performing brain operations on animals have long recognized that mortality was reduced if large lesions were made in separated stages, but the behavioral benefits of multiple-stage lesions were discovered only by chance in the 1940s. HARLOW ADES (1946) was investigating the importance of peristriate cortex in monkeys by performing bilateral ablations of areas 18 and 19. Each animal was trained and tested preoperatively in discriminations of size, shape, and color, and further testing was done postoperatively. In the case of one monkey, the operation had to be interrupted after areas 18 and 19 were removed in one hemisphere. Postoperative retention was perfect after unilateral removal. The second hemisphere was operated 18 days after the first, and again perfect retention was found, whereas the monkeys with one-stage bilateral operations all showed poor retention for all three tasks. Ades and colleagues then tested effects of successive unilateral operations in other cortical areas and found that they spared function in motor cortex (ADES & RAAB, 1946) and in auditory cortex (STEWART & ADES, 1951). In the latter experiment, at least 7 days had to elapse between operations in order to preserve function, but interoperative training did not seem to be necessary.

Investigation of effects of single versus multiple-stage lesions has become an active topic of research in recent years, and the review of FINGER (1978b) cites over 40 studies on this question, mostly from the 1970s. Many factors have been investigated, including these: (a) Duration of interlesion interval. Too short an interval nullifies the benefit of spaced lesions. (b) Size of each lesion. Four-stage removals spaced 3 weeks apart gave better results than two larger lesions spaced 10 weeks apart (STEIN, BUTTERS & ROSEN, 1977). (c) Interoperative testing and training. This has been reported to be helpful in some experiments but not in others; the role of training cannot yet be specified. (d) Interoperative environmental or pharmacological stimulation. Environmental stimulation aids retention, and pharmacological stimulation has been reported in some cases to make up for lack of environmental stimulation.

The animal experiments may help to understand clinical cases such as one described by GESCHWIND (1974, p.489). This patient underwent repeated operations to remove tumor from his temporal lobe. After each operation he became aphasic but each time recovered essentially to normal, even after the last operation when only a thin rim of temporal lobe remained at the base and along the medial surface. This looks like a serial lesion effect but one cannot be certain because an occasional patient recovers from aphasia even after large acute lesions. As GESCHWIND remarks, it would require examination of a number of cases with multiple versus single operations to be certain, and human case reports do not afford such data.

As well as helping to understand why effects of a slowly developing brain lesion may be rather small in view of the amount of tissue destroyed, are there other possible applications to human beings of the findings with the serial-lesion animal model? Here are some possibilities: (a) Although it is infrequent that a therapeutic brain operation can be performed in separated stages rather than at once, when this is possible, multiple-stage operations may result in lesser disability. (b) Perhaps the slow progressive loss of brain cells that occurs during aging can be considered a kind of slowly developing disseminated lesion. The serial-lesion model may help to understand why relatively little functional loss may occur in spite of considerable loss of neurons. (c) But most important are likely to be further contributions of this model to understanding how lesions impair behavior and how recovery occurs. Several hypotheses have been advanced to explain the serial-lesion effect. None seems to be completely satisfactory so far, demonstrating the lack of understanding of these problems, and research continues actively.

C. Secondary and progressive neural degeneration

In some of our experiments involving cortical lesions and differential experience, we have found evidence of both secondary and also progressive loss of cells. Brains with lesions restricted to the occipital cortex were found to have reduced weight and DNA in the rest of the cortex (WILL et al., 1977). This indicated a loss of cells which amounted to about half the loss caused directly by the lesion. Part of the behavioral deficits caused by lesions may be due to this secondary loss of neurons. When we first reported the remote loss, we noted indications that it might be slightly less in EC than in IC rats, but subsequent experiments have shown no significant difference between EC and IC animals in this respect (see Table 4). The further experiments did yield an unexpected finding, however. Table 4 indicates that the secondary loss of cells was somewhat greater in animals sacrificed 100 days after the operation than in those sacrificed 40 days after the operation

Table 4. Percentage losses in weight and total DNA of cortex outside of occipital area, 30 or 90 days after occipital cortex lesions.

Experiment	Age at operation	Postlesion environment	Losses in			
			Tissue weight		Total DNA	
			30 days	90 days	30 days	90 days
A. Larger occipital lesions						
12	32	EC	9.1****	10.5*****	8.0***	9.8****
12	32	IC	8.1****	9.1*****	5.4*	9.0***
15	33	EC	10.6*****	8.3*****	10.2****	7.8****
15	33	IC	6.4**	10.1*****	6.6***	10.6*****
21	59	SC	5.1**	4.9**	5.0**	5.7*
			7.9****	8.6*****	7.4****	8.6****
B. Smaller occipital lesions						
12	32	EC	4.6****	5.3*	4.0***	4.9**
12	32	IC	3.8*	1.3	2.5*	1.0
15	33	EC	2.1	6.4***	1.6	6.5***
15	33	IC	2.5	5.7***	2.1	4.1*
21	59	SC	4.1**	3.0	2.9	5.4
			3.4***	4.3***	2.6**	4.4***

* p < .10, ** p < .05, *** p < .01, **** p < .001

(ROSENZWEIG et al., 1978). Thus it appears that the remote loss of cells increases with time after a localized lesion is made. We are continuing work to define this effect. It suggests that recovery of function may be even more impressive than it appears, if it takes place against a background of progressive loss of brain cells.

The progressive loss of cells remote from the site of the lesion calls to mind an observation of YAKOVLEV reported by GESCHWIND (1974, pp.481–482). YAKOVLEV found that the brain of a patient with a recent prefrontal lobotomy is, except in the immediate vicinity of the lesion, essentially the same as that of a control person. But if quite a few years (say, 20 or more) have elapsed since the lobotomy, then the brain of the patient is markedly diminished. «The longer the time from lobotomy the greater the shrinkage. It seems likely that extensive transsynaptic and transneuronal degeneration is taking place.» Moreover, there is an associated behavioral decline. In the first years after lobotomy, the patients performed as well as controls. Several years later, however, there was a dramatic decline among the operates (HAMLIN, 1970).

The preliminary observations of progressive loss of cells in rats after a localized lesion suggest that this preparation may provide a model for certain human cases, and we plan to look into this question further.

III. Attempts to resolve apparent discrepancies between man and animal in brain-behavior relationships

The basic hypothesis that most cerebral mechanisms of behavior are similar in human beings and in other mammals has so frequently proved correct and is so widely accepted that apparent exceptions have often provided the impetus for research. In some cases this research has led to discoveries of value or of potential value for rehabilitation. Let us consider rather briefly three examples, one involving communication, another concerning memory, and the third having to do with perception.

A. Language in man and in ape

Although language has been held to be unique to human beings, growing knowledge of both the behavioral capacities and the cerebral mechanisms of other primates has led to further consideration of the actual and potential communicative repertories of several primate species (e. g., review or chapter in ALTMANN, 1967; HINDE, 1972; LANCASTER, 1975). It has also been found that the great apes have hemispheric asymmetries similar to those found in human brains; an especially clear example is in the Sylvian fissure which is related to the language region of the human brain (GALABURDA et al., 1978).

Attempts were even made to teach human speech to chimpanzees, but these failed because differences in structure of the mouth and throat preclude the apes from forming human sounds. But it has now been demonstrated that chimpanzees and gorillas are capable of learning arbitrary symbols that stand for nouns, verbs, adjectives, and other parts of speech. In different laboratories, different kinds of symbolic representation have been learned by apes; these symbol systems include American Sign Language for the deaf (GARDNER & GARDNER, 1969; FOUTS, 1975), visual displays activated by keys on a console (RUMBAUGH et al., 1973), and variously shaped and colored metal chips that can be placed on a magnetic board (PREMACK & PREMACK, 1972). The primates have shown themselves capable of asking and answering questions and occasionally of inventing creative combinations of terms. In fact, as this research has advanced, some of the criteria used to distinguish the capacities of animals from those of human beings have had to be abandoned, although substantial differences remain between the communication behavior of the trained animals and human language (LIMBER, 1977).

Some of this research, in which the attempt was made to extend the human model to animals, has now yielded an unexpected application to human patients. DAVID PREMACK, a psychologist who had taught a chimpanzee to manipulate colored chips to express rather complicated concepts, later took part in a successful attempt to re-open communication channels to severely aphasic patients by similar techniques (GLASS, GAZZANIGA & PREMACK, 1973). Seven globally asphasic patients with damage to the left hemisphere were given training in selection and manipulation of cut-out paper symbols to represent objects and relations. In hindsight it does not seem surprising that most of the patients were able to learn a system originally devised for nonhuman primates. Individuals varied, of course, progressing to levels that ranged from expressions of object relations to making simple statements of action. The investigators concluded that despite massive loss of language, globally aphasic patients retain a rich conceptual system and at least some capacity for symbolization and primitive linguistic functions. As well as providing these patients some possibilities for communication, the training afforded a fuller assessment of their capacities than did conventional methods of testing.

Other attempts are also being made to aid human beings whose language is impaired or deficient by using systems designed or employed to allow communication with apes. Thus, attempts are being made to teach American Sign Language to mute autistic children, and a positive preliminary report has been published (BONVILLIAN & NELSON, 1976). The report describes a mute autistic boy who learned sign language. Analysis of the signs and sign combinations that he produced over a 6-month period indicated the presence of a full range of semantic relations. Moreover, during the time he learned to sign, both scores on a concept test and social behavior improved. The extent of the boy's linguistic and behavioral progress exceeded that usually reported for mute autistic children, and further work is being done in this direction. A recent newspaper report indicated that the original console and computer used by RUMBAUGH at Tulane for communication with chimpanzees have been given to an institution for retarded children. A few severely retarded children are reported to be showing considerable progress with this system. For example, an 18-year-old girl who had a vocabulary of only 11 words was reported to have gained a vocabulary of 100 words on the machine; she also showed improvement in behavior and motivation. The kinds of brain deficits that are present in autism or in most cases of mental retardation have not yet been identified, but these examples indicate new possibilities for rehabilitation, derived from an animal model.

While this application may seem rather limited, the discoveries about communicative abilities in apes may lead to further advances in our understanding of the cerebral mechanisms of language and of possible therapies for aphasia. In regard to cerebral mechanisms, the brains of chimpanzees are now being used for detailed mapping of connections among cortical regions that serve language functions in human beings. If the chimpanzee is an appropriate model in this regard, then such anatomical studies can supply valuable information that cannot now be obtained directly from human brains. Of course, as we will discuss further in the final section, the model cannot simply be assumed to be equivalent to the human brain, and all proposed extrapolations must be subjected to searching tests.

B. Memory deficits resulting from lesions of medial temporal lobe

In the 1960s an apparently major discrepancy was pointed out between the results of pathology in the medial area of the temporal lobe in human patients and experimental lesions made to study the syndrome in animal subjects. It had been found in the 1950s that bilateral destruction in the medial temporal lobe in patients led to the inability to form new long-term memories although short-term memories could be formed and earlier memories remained intact. Such cases have occurred in surgical removal of the hippocampus in epileptic or brain-injured patients, as in the case of H.M. operated on by SCOVILLE in 1953 for the relief of epilepsy and studied over many years by MILNER and associates (SCOVILLE & MILNER, 1957; MILNER, CORKIN & TEUBER, 1968; MILNER, 1972). Bilateral destruction in the hippocampal region by an attack of herpes encephalitis was also found to lead to similar defects of memory (ROSE & SYMONDS, 1960; STARR & PHILLIPS, 1970).

It was concluded that the memory impairment was caused by damage to the hippocampus, but destruction of the hippocampus in experimental animals was found not to prevent the formation of lasting memories in a wide variety of behavioral tests (DOUGLAS, 1967; KIMBLE, 1968; ISAACSON, 1972). Attempts to resolve the apparent lack of correspondence between results of human and animal hippocampal lesions have led to a number of creative interpretations and also to some important behavioral and neurological findings.

Of course, it could have been concluded the hippocampus performs different functions in man and in animal so that correspondence is not to be expected. There has not been much enthusiasm for this interpretation, however, and further observations indicate that it is not necessary to adopt this conclusion.

Quite a different interpretation is that the main deficit of the hippocampal patients is one of retrieval rather than of memory storage. Experiments with hippocampectomized animals revealed that they had greater difficulty than normals in abandoning earlier learning or strategies; they showed greater interference of earlier learning on later tasks (e.g., DOUGLAS, 1967; KIMBLE, 1968). The persistence of response in the animal subjects accorded with an observation made by WARRINGTON and WEISKRANTZ (1968) concerning verbal learning in amnesic patients. The patients seemed unable to learn even simple lists of words after several repetitions. But as they were given one list after another, the experimenters began to recognize that many of the wrong responses seemed familiar. Analysis showed that many of the wrong responses were actually words from earlier lists in the experiment. Thus the words were being stored but were emerging at the wrong time. Further work showed that providing cues at the time of recall could substantially improve the performance of amnesic patients (WEISKRANTZ & WARRINGTON, 1975). Thus the defect may be more in the retrieval than in the storage of memories. WEISKRANTZ (1977, p.438) concludes with satisfaction that there no longer need be «any embarrassment over being unable to find a blockade of input into longterm memory in the animal, because there is no such blockade in man either» as a consequence of hippocampal destruction. In line with this conclusion, a number of investigators have shown that amnesic patients and others who suffer from problems of memory can be aided both by using strategies of encoding and by cuing at retrieval (e.g., SIGNORET & LHERMITTE, 1976; POON, in press), and such methods can undoubtedly be employed more thoroughly for the benefit of many who suffer from impairments of memory.

But not all workers in this area are satisfied that the retrieval-impairment hypothesis accounts for all aspects of amnesia or that it closes completely the gap between symptoms in humans and in animals with temporal lobe damage. Although the retrieval impairment hypothesis can account for a number of observations and suggests useful techniques for recovering memories, ROZIN (1976) has pointed out that it does not account for certain salient phenomena. If the deficit is one of retrieval, how is it that memories acquired before brain damage can be retrieved readily whereas only those acquired later are difficult to retrieve without special cuing? Also, amnesic patients show a striking lack of familiarity for postlesion memories even after they are retrieved, and this is not explained by the retrieval hypothesis. Such a lack of familiarity is not, of course, tested in animal subjects. We simply note whether an animal subject responds correctly or not, without inquiring whether the stimuli seem familiar or about any aspects of the animal's conscious awareness. Perhaps such observations could be made with apes that have been trained to communicate, but I do not know of any plans at present to subject such animals to brain lesions for experimental purposes. (Ethical problems involved in such experiments will be referred to later in this paper.) The fact that we observe behavior in animals but typically ask for verbal reports from patients is also responsible, in part at least, for the apparent discrepancy to be discussed in the section C below.

A very different approach followed recently by HOREL (1978) has been to re-examine critically whether the site of the lesion responsible for the memory deficits is in fact the hippocampus or some other structure in the ventromedial quadrant of the temporal lobe. From his scrutiny of the literature,

HOREL concludes that the critical site is probably the temporal stem, that is, the albal stalk that carries the afferent and efferent connections of temporal cortex and amygdala but that does not carry connections of the hippocampus. The position of the temporal stem (see Fig.2) makes it vulnerable to the surgical approach that was used in the human medial temporal lobectomies. Furthermore, when the stem was sectioned in monkeys without damaging the hippocampus, severe deficits in learning and retention were produced (HOREL & MISANTONE, 1974, 1976). Among the connections of the temporal lobe whose damage might be responsible for the memory defect, HOREL emphasizes those to the medial magnocellular part of the medialis dorsalis nucleus of the thalamus (see Fig.2). Pathology in this nucleus has been strongly implicated in the memory defects that occur in Korsakoff's syndrome (VICTOR, ADAMS & COLLINS, 1971). If Horel's hypothesis is confirmed, it will have important implications for directing neurosurgery in the temporal lobe so as to reduce the possibilities of impairing memory. It will also serve to re-

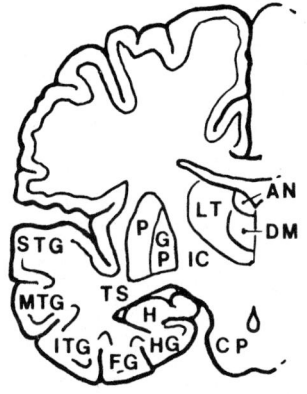

Figure 2. Coronal sections of brain, with labelling of temporal lobe and neighboring structures. AN, anterior nuclear group of thalamus; DP, cerebral peduncle; DM, dorsomedial nucleus; FG, fusiform gyrus of temporal lobe; GP, globus pallidus; H, hippocampus; HG, hippocampal gyrus, IC, internal capsule; ITG, inferior temporal gyrus; LT, lateral thalamus; MTG, middle temporal gyrus; P. putamen; STG, superior temporal gyrus; TS, temporal stem.

orient thinking about the neural circuits involved in memory. And it will provide further justification for use of animal models to study mechanisms of the human brain.

C. Effects of lesions of visual cortex in man and animal

Evidence from over half a century of research has shown that damage to the striate cortex (area 17) in man produces severe blindness, whereas the monkey with similar damage conserves considerable visual capacity. Human patients without striate cortex have been reported to detect, at the most, vigorous movement or abrupt changes in illumination. In contrast, as programs of testing animals advanced, progressively greater capacities were revealed in monkeys even after complete removal of primary visual cortex. Not only light flux but also simple patterns and location of events in the visual field could be discriminated by the brain-lesioned monkeys.

As in the example of memory and temporal lobe damage discussed in the preceding section, the apparent discrepancy in visual capacity of man and monkey after damage to visual cortex could be taken in different ways. It could be interpreted as revealing a fundamental difference in brain-behavior relations in human beings and nonhuman primates. Or it could serve as a challenge to investigate more thoroughly the visual capacities of brain-injured patients by employing behavioral techniques similar to those used with nonverbal animals. A few investigators have taken up this challenge.

Patients with discrete destruction of primary visual cortex are rather rare, but a few of them have been studied in some detail in the last few years. The patient studied by WEISKRANTZ and his colleagues in England provides an example (SANDERS et al., 1974; WEISKRANTZ et al., 1974; WEISKRANTZ, 1977). This patient had a small tumor removed from his right calcarine fissure, and on subsequent routine testing he appeared to be completely blind in the left-half fields of both eyes, even to intense lights. There was a small crescent of fuzzy vision in the upper peripheral part of the field, so further detailed testing was confined to the lower quadrant. In the first experimental tests the subject was asked to reach out and touch the position on a screen at which a visual stimulus was projected briefly in the blind field. This is the same sort of task that monkeys were trained to perform in order to obtain rewards. It seems like an odd task to ask of a person who says that he can't see in the region being tested, but the subject was asked to «guess» where the stimulus might be on each trial, and he cooperated. It soon became apparent that he was able to locate stimuli quite accurately. When the results of these trials were shown to the subject after several hours of testing, he was astonished. Later he described «feelings» that something might be present, but he consistently refused to call this the «seeing» that he had in his right-half fields. Later this subject was asked to guess if the stimulus was a horizontal or a vertical line, or X versus 0. He showed about 75% accuracy with stimuli 12° in size and even greater accuracy with larger stimuli. He could discriminate whether lines or a homogeneous field appeared in an aperture, although he denied seeing even the bright aperture in which the test stimuli appeared. His acuity as measured in this way was less than 2 minutes of arc. The subject was not using his sighted fields to accomplish these performances; he reported quickly if even a faint stimulus appeared at the edge of his intact field.

The investigators termed this capacity «blindsight.» The patient does not perceive yet he performs visual discriminations. This distinction suggests issues at both applied and theoretical levels.

Considering the possibility of applications of «blindsight», could patients develop both the acuity and the confidence in this type of vision to be able to use it in daily life? MOHLER & WURTZ (1977) have found that in monkeys with lesions in part of the striate cortex, the ability to detect a spot of light in the «blind» area increased with training. Moreover, the training was specific, since the areas of the visual field that received practice recovered more rapidly than those that were not practiced. HUMPHREY (1970) has reported that a monkey with complete destruction of striate cortex not only learned to discriminate targets but also used vision to avoid obstacles. Active training rather than imposition of stimuli upon a passive animal appears to be necessary for improvement of visual discrimination after lesions of striate cortex (COWEY, 1967). The critical features of this «behavioral therapy» are not yet known, but HUMPHREY and WEISKRANTZ (1967) note that one important aspect seems to be the arranging of visual events in the animal's environment in such a way that he can relate them to distinctive features of tactile-kinesthetic space and obtain rapid and reliable feedback from those features. The experimenters reported that at the outset of such training, the animal seems to discover that it possesses a viable visual space, and after this discovery is made, then performance can improve rather rapidly. There are many kinds of performance that people carry out on the basis of barely detectable or even subliminal stimuli. Further research is needed to determine whether training of blindsight can be used in practical situations by blind people.

It should be emphasized that the discovery of blindsight occurred because investigators familiar with brain-behavior relations in animals were intrigued and concerned about an apparent discrepancy between the human and the animal relations in this case. Using behavioral methods devised for nonverbal animal subjects, they discovered unexpected capacities in brain-damaged human beings. Routine clinical testing methods that rely on patients to tell us what they are able to see or do may fall far short of revealing the full capabilities of the patients.

Presumably in the present case the discrimination was carried out by circuits that include the superior colliculus. Evidence for this was obtained by MOHLER and WURTZ (1977). They found that if they made lesions in appropriate areas of both the striate cortex and the superior colliculus, the monkey was unable to recover any visual discrimination in the affected part of the field. It appears then that the circuit involving the superior colliculus has information-processing capacity and adequate connections to motor controls but is only weakly connected to parts of the brain required for conscious awareness. Such clues should be helpful toward further elucidation of brain circuits required for consciousness as distinct for those required for behavioral discrimination.

While we do not have direct tests for animal consciousness, it may nevertheless be possible to carry out some of this research with animal subjects. Thus, it has been reported that monkeys with striate cortex lesions seemed to suffer from agnosia since they discriminated forms but did not appear to recognize objects (HUMPHREY, 1970). This conclusion was based on observations that although the monkey could reach for objects and avoid obstacles, it appeared to show no interest in the sight of a tasty carrot and no fear of a toy snake held in front of it.

When a patient with brain injury has an area of the visual field that is blind by perimetric testing, this does not necessarily mean that all of the cells in the cortical projection area corresponding to the deficit have been destroyed; training can sometimes produce restitution of function even though the blindness has persisted for months or even years (ZIHL & VON CRAMON, 1979). Especially when there was a gradual transition between the scotoma and normal parts of the visual field, training to discriminate intensity differences around the borders of the scotoma led to its shrinkage. Although training was restricted to contrast sensitivity, improvement was also found in visual acuity, critical flicker fusion, and perception of color. The improvement did not occur spontaneously but only during training periods. In some cases the training resulted in remarkable improvement in behavioral capacities. One patient had only a very small intact part of his visual field and was functionally blind for more than 4 years; he found his way around with acoustic and tactile cues. During a few months of training, the upper left quadrant was restored so that the patient now walks using visual cues and can read a newspaper.

IV. Animal models: Problems and prospects

The preceding pages have offered a small selection from a large literature bearing on animal models for brain mechanisms of behavior in human beings; the attempt was made to chose some examples of possible relevance to recovery of

157

function following brain injury. Other chapters in this book present other examples of animal models for aspects of rehabilitation. Some of these examples may prove to be useful and to increase our understanding of human beings – and of animals. If put into practice, these ideas should have beneficial effects and help men and women to perform nearer to their full capacities. Some examples may be faulty and lead to confusion; if put into practice these may limit or even impair the behavior of individuals and may have undesirable social consequences.

Are there criteria by which we can usually distinguish between fruitful and misleading animal models? And what tests should be applied to results or inferences drawn from investigation of models?

A. Criteria for selecting animal models

There are several criteria for choosing adequate animal models to throw light on brain-behavior relations in human beings, and different criteria may point to different choices, so compromises are often necessary. Let us list and examine some major criteria that have been proposed:

(a) The model must exhibit behavior that shows functional properties similar to those that are of concern in the human being. For example, if neural mechanisms of learning are to be studied (and learning is certainly involved in some cases of recovery), then the model organism should exhibit the main varieties of learning that people show. (Some proposed invertebrate models show habituation but not classical or instrumental conditioning.) In order to apply this criterion, the investigator needs to know a good deal about the behavior of the animal and also of the human being.

(b) The model should use (or at least be presumed to use) the same causal mechanisms that hold (or are presumed to hold) for the human. Following this criterion, one would not select an amphibian which readily regenerates nerves as a model for recovery of function in mammals which do not show much regeneration.

(c) It is sometimes held that one should go beyond criteria *a* and *b* and choose a model as similar to *homo sapiens* as possible, behaviorally, anatomically, and physiologically. In line with this thinking, the primates have often been considered to be the models of choice. But WARREN and KOLB (1978) have suggested instead the following formulation: The model should be within the same taxon as man in regard to the behavior and neural mechanism that are being considered. That is, in the case of a behavior and its neural mechanism that are in common for all mammals, any member of the class of mammals can serve as a model. For a behavior and neural mechanism that are found only in primates, any primate will be an adequate model. For any behavior and mechanism that can be determined to be unique to man, no other species can serve as a model. WARREN and KOLB point out that many more neural mechanisms are in common for the class of mammals than was believed only a few years ago when evidence seemed to support the concept of encephalization of function within the mammalian class. While this implies that there is much generality of brain-behavior relations among mammals, it does not mean that differences in behavior and in brain structure among mammalian species can be neglected.

(d) The model should be chosen so that the process of interest can be studied in as direct and simple a way as possible. This is a reason why research on genetic mechanisms in the bacterium *E. coli* was so successful.

(e) Animals of the species chosen should be abundant, inexpensive, easy to handle, and breed well in captivity, so that well-designed experiments with adequate numbers of subject can be carried out readily.

It is apparent that in practice some of these criteria will run counter to others. For example, while the use of primates is desirable for their similarity to man, they are not abundant or inexpensive. In fact, an attempt is now being made in the United States to revise the requirement that certain tests of drugs be performed on monkeys, because rodents are an adequate model for these tests and are much less expensive. While a chimpanzee that had been trained to use sign language might from some points of view make an excellent subject for study of effects of experimental brain damage on language, the great expense of training such subjects makes it unlikely that they will be used to investigate effects of brain damage. And even if expense were not a barrier, questions are being raised about the ethics of keeping animals confined if they are capable of language-like behavior. Let us turn briefly to this ethical concern.

Research using animals models for human behavior has had the paradoxical result that the demonstrated similarities between animals and human beings are now being used to support the claim that there are «animal rights» analogous to «human rights.» Here are a few examples of this trend which appears to be growing: A professor of philosophy, PETER SINGER, has attempted to discuss the issues of human treatment of nonhumans on political and moral bases in his book, «Animal liberation» (1975). The astronomer and science popularizer CARL SAGAN asks the following question in his recent book on evolution of the mind – a book that draws heavily on studies of animal brain and behavior: «Why, exactly, all over the civilized world, in virtually every major city, are apes in prison?» (1977, p. 121). The *Christian Science Monitor* ran a series of three articles on research with laboratory animals, March 8–10, 1978; it concluded with recommendations for tighter legal controls on such research, development of courses dealing with moral and ethical issues involved in animal experimentation, and research to develop alternatives to animal testing in the screening of drugs and products. Pressures in these directions are likely to become of increasing concern to investigators who use animals for the purposes of lessening human suffering and rehabilitating brain-injured patients.

The criterion of selecting a model that allows most direct study of a process may indicate a different choice than would be made on the criterion of closeness of relationship to man. Thus, in the study of neural processes of learning and memory, there is much current research on relatively simple animals like the sea hare, *Aplysia*. KANDEL (1976), one of the chief investigators of these models, has defined the advantages of the simple-systems approach using invertebrate preparations. Although the behavior of these systems is limited and thus these models do not meet the first criterion listed above, KANDEL argues that complex «emergent» properties of the behavior of higher animals are best approached in terms of the ability of interacting systems of cells to manifest properties that could not or might not be readily inferred from studies of cells in isolation; programmatically, the study of small circuits of cells comes first and should afford a secure basis for all the rest. Other investigators believe that more useful models for neural processes in learning are to be discovered in certain relatively simple circuits that are found in mammalian brains.

Whatever order or family of animals one chooses for the purpose of providing suitable models for neural plasticity in human beings, it is certain to be some type of animal subject because the experimental procedures required in this research are not kinds to which one would want to subject people. At the same time that I drafted this paper, EDWARD BENNETT and I wrote a chapter «How plastic is the nervous system?» for a book entitled *Comprehensive handbook of behavioral medicine* (ROSENZWEIG & BENNETT, in press). Needless to say, the examples of neural plasticity, which were meant to stimulate the thought processes of therapists, were almost all drawn from animal research – largely, but not exclusively, research done with mammalian subjects. One criterion calls for knowing both the model species and the human being very well in regard to the behavior being studied, and this could also be extended to the brain mechanisms of the behavior. But in fact it is precisely because we do not know enough about human beings in certain regards that we find animal models helpful. In respect to this criterion, those whose primary concern is rehabilitation differ from those whose primary concern is in comparison among species. For the student of comparative behavior and of comparative brain mechanisms, all species may be of equal importance. But clinicians and investigators of recovery of function are interested in animal models only insofar as they may contribute to understanding of human behavior and its neural bases. For example, KANDEL, who came to his studies of invertebrate preparations from a medical background, states that the invertebrate research would lose much of its interest and value if it were not useful in providing a basis for the study of vertebrate and eventually of human behavior (1976, p.652). On the contrary, some other investigators of neural mechanisms of learning and memory in invertebrates (e.g., Davis, 1976; Krasne, 1976) believe that these studies would be of value even if they had no application to human beings, although they argue that given the conservatism of nature, the findings concerning neural mechanisms of invertebrates are likely to apply to other orders as well.

But even if the proper study of mankind is man, there is value in objective study of animal behavior because of the stimulating and original questions it suggests about human behavior. Apparent discrepancies between human and animal brain-behavior relations have provided the impetus for many enlightening investigations, some with potentials for application to rehabilitation, as was illustrated in part III above. Some of the most interesting work of this sort is being done by investigators who study both human and animal subjects, as in some of the examples noted above.

B. Testing conclusions drawn from animal models

However carefully we apply criteria to select suitable animal models for a particular problem, and however skillfully we conduct the research, there is still no guarantee that the conclusions drawn from the experimental results will be useful in solving the problem. Any particular finding can be interpreted in terms of a large number of hypotheses – the number being limited only by the inventiveness of researchers and theoreticians. To winnow out viable interpretations and discard false hypotheses, systematic application of «strong inference» is a powerful technique (Platt, 1964).

The utility of an apparently productive finding can be determined only by attempting to put it into practice. Here there is an obvious advantage for those investigators who are participating in work with both animal and human subjects and who can turn readily from experimental research to tests of application. But for most investigators who do not play such a dual role, it is important at least to be conversant with the other side of the coin – on the one side the problems and challenges of recovery of function and rehabilitation, and on the other, the techniques and resources of research with animal models.

It is difficult to apply the criterion that the animal model should be within the same taxon as man for the behavior and neural mechanism being considered, because we often lack the information that would be needed for a rigorous decision on these grounds. Therefore we often have to proceed in a «bootstrap» manner, using a model that seems plausible based on the best current knowledge, then attempting to apply the conclusions to man and using the success or failure of the attempt to help determine the limits within which such models should be chosen in the future. A review of such attempts could also be used to assess the overall value of the method of employing animal models as it has been practiced.

As stated at the outset, I have not tried here to compile a substantial number of attempts to employ animal models and then to assess the proportions of success or failure. That would be a herculean task. Therefore the following statements about the degree of success of animal models for brain-behavior relations in different behavioral fields are simply impressions derived from knowledge of a small sample of investigations of this sort.

First, the neural mechanisms for many aspects of sensation and perception have been clearly demonstrated to be the same for man and primates (and in many cases for other mammals as well). As examples of this, BENTON (1978) has traced the history of research on representation of vision in the cerebral cortex and on the method of double sensory stimulation in detecting unilateral lesions. We have shown above that even an apparent discrepancy between the role of primary visual cortex in monkey and in man has turned out, upon more searching investigation, not to be real (Section IIIC). Second, the cerebral motor circuits are also similar in man and other primates, although the upright posture of man necessitates certain differences. Third, the mechanisms of biological motivational systems such as hunger and thirst are also likely to be similar in man and other mammals, although we are less sure because this area is less far advanced than those of perception and motor functions.

Fourth, social behavior is an area in which it has been more difficult to employ animal models for human behavior than in the cases mentioned in the last paragraph. In social behavior we include such examples as communication, aggression, socio-sexual behavior, and group structures. A good deal of research in this area has been summarized and discussed by HINDE (1974). Animal behavior is exceedingly diverse, so that it is easy to select striking examples to bolster almost any ethical, social or political argument, especially if exception or contrary examples are neglected. Examples of such controversies are the arguments concerning the inevitability of aggression, as stated by some ethologists, and the application to human society of the principles of «sociobiology.» Other examples somewhat closer to our present concern can also be mentioned. The distress of infant rhesus macaques upon separation from the mother has been used as a model for the «anaclitic depression» of institutionalized children. But while pig-tailed macaque infants show responses similar to those of rhesus monkeys when the mother is removed from the group, bonnet macaques and squirrel monkeys show little distress when the mother is removed, partly because the infant-mother bonds are less exclusive in these latter species, and partly because other females in the troop are more likely to look after the infant (KAUFMAN & ROSENBLUM, 1969; ROSENBLUM, 1971). Which, if any, of these species is an appropriate model for the human case? Animal models have also been proposed for many aspects of human sexual behavior, including homosexual behavior. BEACH (in press) has criticized an attempt to use a rodent model for human homosexual behavior and has suggested that study of primates is more likely to provide a suitable model. WASHBURN (1978) has pointed out that the nature of ape behavior and its relation to human behavior was debated for more than a hundred years before reliable data began to be gathered, mostly in the last decade.

For example, the idea that sexual attraction is responsible for existence of the social group in nonhuman primates and in human societies was long propounded by social theorists and has been restated recently by some sociobiologists, but WASH-BURN shows that the social attraction theory of society does not fit the data, even in the case of the apes.

Aspects of social behavior important to rehabilitation include communication and social motivation. Communication is relevant to rehabilitation in many ways – as an area for therapy (as in aphasia), in the evaluation and assessment of impairment, and in therapeutic attempts (as in teaching strategies to improve learning and memory). Motivation has been stressed by Professor GLEES at this symposium as well as by many students of rehabilitation. Professor GLEES and others have employed animal models to investigate this factor in recovery of function, but further research and definition of appropriate models can probably still teach us much more about the use of motivation to obtain the fullest possible rehabilitation.

It seems appropriate to conclude this paper with a paragraph that HARRY HARLOW wrote for an article on the related topic of generalization of behavioral data between nonhuman and human animals:

Basically the problems of generalization of behavioral data between species are simple – one cannot generalize, but one must. If the competent do not with to generalize, the incompetent will fill the field. (HARLOW, GLUCK & SUOMI, 1972, p. 716.)

Bibliography

ADES, H. W.: Effects of extirpation of parastriate cortex on learned visual discriminations in monkeys. J. Neuropath. & Exp. Neurol. 5, 60–66, 1946.

ADES, H. W., RAAB, D. H.: Recovery of motor function after two stage extirpation of area 4 in monkeys (Macaca mulatta). J. Neurophysiol. 9, 55–60, 1946.

ALTMANN, S. A. (Ed.): Social Communication Among Primates. University of Chicago Press, Chicago 1967; p. 392.

ALTSCHULER, R. A.: Changes in hippocampal synaptic density with increased learning experience in the rat. Soc. Neurosci. Abstrs. 2, 438, 1976.

BEACH, F.A.: Animal models for human sexuality. In: Whelan, J. (Ed.): Sex, Hormones and Behaviour, Ciba Foundation Symposium 62. London, Ciba Foundation (in press).

BENNETT, E.L.: Cerebral effects of differential experience and training. In: Rosenzweig, M.R., Bennett, E.L. (Eds.): Neural Mechanisms of Learning and Memory. MIT Press, Cambridge 1976; pp.279–287.

BENNETT, E.L., DIAMOND, M.C., KRECH, D., ROSENZWEIG, M.R.: Chemical and anatomical plasticity of brain. Science *146,* 610–619, 1964.

BENNETT, E.L., ROSENZWEIG, M.R., MORIMOTO, H., HEBERT, M.: Maze training alters brain weights and cortical RNA/DNA. Behav. & Neural Biol. (in press).

BENNETT, E.L., ROSENZWEIG, M.R., WU, S.Y.C.: Excitant and depressant drugs modulate effects of environment on brain weight and cholinesterase. Psychopharmacologia *33,* 309–328, 1973.

BENTON, A.: The interplay of experimental and clinical approaches in brain lesion research. In: Finger, S. (Ed.): Recovery from Brain Damage. Plenum Press, New York 1978; pp.49–68.

BONVILLIAN, J.D., NELSON, K.E.: Sign language acquisition in a mute autistic boy. J.Speech & Hearing Disorders *41,* 339–347, 1976.

BRUDNY, J., KOREIN, J., GRYNBAUM, B.B., FRIEDMANN, L.W., WEINSTEIN, S., SACHS-FRANKEL, G., BELANDRES, P.V.: EMG feedback therapy: Review of treatment of 114 patients. Archives Phys.Med.Rehab. *57,* 55–61, 1976.

COWEY, A.: Perimetric study of field defects in monkeys after cortical and retinal ablations. Quarterly J.Exp.Psychol. *19,* 232–245, 1967.

DAVENPORT, J.W.: Environment as therapy for brain effects of endocrine dysfunction. In: Walsh, R.N., Greenough, W.T. (Eds.): Environments as Therapy for Brain Dysfunction. Plenum Press, New York 1976; pp.71–114.

DAVIS, W.J.: Plasticity in the invertebrates. In: Rosenzweig, M.R., Bennett, E.L. (Eds.): Neural Mechanism of Learning and Memory. MIT Press, Cambridge 1976; pp.430–462.

DIAMOND, M.C., INGHAM, C.A., JOHNSON, R.E., BENNETT, E.L., ROSENZWEIG, M.R.: Effects of environment on morphology of rat cerebral cortex and hippocampus. J.Neurobiol. *7,* 75–85, 1976.

DIAMOND, M.C., KRECH, D., ROSENZWEIG, M.R.: The effects of an enriched environment on the histology of the rat cerebral cortex. J.Comp.Neurol. *123,* 111–119, 1964.

DIAMOND, M.C., LAW, F., RHODES, H., LINDNER, B., ROSENZWEIG, M.R., KRECH, D., BENNETT, E.L.: Increases in cortical depth and glia numbers in rats subjected to enriched environment. J.Comp.Neurol. *128,* 117–125, 1966.

DIAMOND, M.C., LINDNER, B., JOHNSON, R., BENNETT, E.L., ROSENZWEIG, M.R.: Differences in occipital cortical synapses from environmentally enriched, impoverished, and standard colony rats. J.Neurosci.Res. *1,* 109–119, 1975.

DOUGLAS, R.J.: The hippocampus and behavior. Psychol.Bull. *67,* 416–442, 1967.

166

FERCHMIN, P.A., ETEROVIĆ, V.A., CAPUTTO, R.: Studies of brain weight and RNA content after short periods of exposure to environmental complexity. Brain Res. *20,* 49–57, 1970.

FINGER, S. (Ed.): Recovery from Brain Damage. Plenum Press, New York 1978a; p.423.

FINGER, S.: Lesion momentum and behavior. In: Finger, S. (Ed.): Recovery from Brain Damage. Plenum Press, New York 1978b; pp.135–164.

FLOETER, M.K., GREENOUGH, W.T., SACKETT, G.P.: Cerebellar plasticity: Modification of dendritic branching by differential rearing in monkeys. Soc.Neurosci.Abstrs. *4,* 471, 1978.

FOUTS, R.S.: Acquisition and testing of gestural signs in four young chimpanzees. Science *180,* 978–980, 1975.

FRANZ, S.I.: On the functions of the cerebrum: The frontal lobes in relation to the production and retention of simple sensory-motor habits. Am.J. Physiol. *8,* 1–22, 1902.

FRANZ, S.I.: Autobiography. In: Murchison, C. (Ed.): A History of Psychology in Autobiography, vol.2. Clark University Press, Worcester, Massachusetts 1932; pp.89–113.

GALABURDA, A.M., LeMAY, M., KEMPER, T.L., GESCHWIND, N.: Right-left asymmetries in the brain. Science *199,* 852–856, 1978.

GARDNER, R.A., GARDNER, P.T.: Teaching sign language to a chimpanzee. Science *165,* 664–672, 1969.

GELLER, E.: Some observations on the effects of environmental complexity and isolation on biochemical ontogeny. In: Sterman, M.B., McGinty, D.J., Adinolfi, A.M. (Eds.): Brain Development and Behavior. Academic Press, New York 1971; pp.277–296.

GESCHWIND, N.: Late changes in the nervous system: An overview. In: Stein, D.G., Rosen, J.J., Butters, N. (Eds.): Plasticity and Recovery of Function in the Central Nervous System. Academic Press, New York 1974; pp.467–508.

GLASS, A.V., GAZZANIGA, M.S., PREMACK, D.: Artificial language training in global aphasics. Neuropsychologia *11,* 95–103, 1973.

GLOBUS, A., ROSENZWEIG, M.R., BENNETT, E.L., DIAMOND, M.C.: Effects of differential experience on dendritic spine counts. J.Comp.Physiol. Psychol. *82,* 175–181, 1973.

GREENOUGH, W.T.: Enduring brain effects of differential experience and training. In: Rosenzweig, M.R., Bennett, E.L. (Eds.): Neural Mechanisms of Learning and Memory. MIT Press, Cambridge 1976; pp.255–278.

GREENOUGH, W.T., FASS, B., DeVOOGD, T.: The influence of experience on recovery following brain damage in rodents: Hypotheses based on developmental research. In: Walsh, R.N., Greenough, W.T. (Eds.): Environments as Therapy for Brain Dysfunction. Plenum Press, New York 1976; pp.10–50.

GREENOUGH, W.T., JURASKA, J.M.: Can we predict behavior from environmentally induced changes in the brain? In: Hahn, M., Jensen, C., Dudek, B. (Eds.): Development and Evolution of Brain Size: Behavioral Implications. Academic Press, New York, in press.

167

HAMLIN, R.M.: Intellectual functions 14 years after frontal lobe surgery. Cortex *6*, 299–307, 1970.

HANIN, I., USDIN, E. (Eds.): Animal Models in Psychiatry and Neurology. Pergamon Press, New York 1977; p.499.

HARLOW, H.F., GLUCK, J.P., SUOMI, S.J.: Generalization of behavioral data between nonhuman and human animals. Am.Psychologist *27*, 709–716, 1972.

HINDE, R.A. (Ed.): Non-verbal Communication. England, Cambridge 1972; p.441.

HINDE, R.A.: Biological Bases of Human Social Behaviour. McGraw-Hill Book Company, New York 1974; p.462.

HOOPER, F.: Rehabilitation of the patient with acquired brain damage. Aust. J.Hum.Commun.Disorders *5*, 7–22, 1977.

HOREL, J.A.: The neuroanatomy of amnesia: A critique of the hippocampal memory hypothesis. Brain *101*, 403–445, 1978.

HOREL, J.A., MISANTONE, L.G.: The Klüver-Bucy syndrome produced by destroying temporal neocortex or amygdala. Brain Res. (Amsterdam) *42*, 101–112, 1974.

HUMPHREY, N.K.: What the frog's eye tells the monkey's brain. Brain.Behav. & Evol. *3*, 324–337, 1970.

HUMPHREY, N.K., WEISKRANTZ, L.: Vision in monkeys after removal of striate cortex. Nature *215*, 595–597, 1967.

KANDEL, E.R.: Cellular Basis of Behavior, An Introduction to Behavioral Neurobiology. W.H.Freeman and Company, San Francisco 1976; p.727.

KATZ, H.B.: Influences of undernutrition on learning performance: A motivational analysis of maze studies. Doctoral dissertation, University of California, Berkeley, 1977.

KAUFMAN, I.C., ROSENBLUM, L.A.: Effects of separation from mother on the emotional behavior of infant monkeys. Ann. N.Y. Acad.Sci. *159*, 681–695, 1969.

KIMBLE, D.P.: Hippocampus and internal inhibition. Psychol.Bull. *70*, 285–295, 1968.

KRASNE, F.B.: Invertebrate systems as a means of gaining insight into the nature of learning and memory. In: Rosenzweig, M.R., Bennett, E.L. (Eds.): Neural Mechanisms of Learning and Memory. MIT Press, Cambridge 1976; pp.401–429.

LANCASTER, J.B.: Primate Behavior and the Emergence of Human Culture. Holt, Rinehart and Winston, New York 1975; p.98.

LIMBER, J.: Language in child and chimp? Am.Psychologist *32*, 280–295, 1977.

LIPTON, M.A., DiMASCIO, A., KILLAM, K.F. (Eds.): Psychopharmacology: A Generation of Progress. Raven Press, New York 1978; p.1731.

MEYER, P.M., HOREL, J.A., MEYER, D.R.: Effects of dl-amphetamine upon placing responses in neodecorticate cats. J.Comp.Physiol.Psychol. *56*, 402–404, 1963.

MILLER, N.E.: Biofeedback and visceral learning. Ann.Rev.Psychol. *29*, 373–404, 1978.

MILNER, B.: Disorders of learning and memory after temporal lobe lesions in man. Clin. Neurosurg. *19*, 421–446, 1972.

MILNER, B., CORKIN, S., TEUBER, H.-L.: Further analysis of the hippocampal amnesic syndrome: 14 year follow-up study of H.M. Neurophysiologia *6*, 215–234, 1968.

MOHLER, C.W., WURTZ, R.H.: Role of striate cortex and superior colliculus in visual guidance of saccadic eye movements in monkeys. J. Neurophysiol. *40*, 74–94, 1977.

MØLLGAARD, K., DIAMOND, M.C., BENNETT, E.L., ROSENZWEIG, M.R., LINDNER, B.: Quantitative synaptic changes with differential experience in rat brain. Internat. J. Neurosci. *2*, 113–128, 1971.

MORIMOTO, H., FERCHMIN, P.A., BENNETT, E.L.: Spectrophotometric analysis of RNA and DNA using cetyltrimethylammonium bromide. Analytical Biochem. *62*, 436–448, 1974.

MORRISON, H., MCKINNEY, W.T.: Environments of dysfunction: The relevance of primate animal models. In: Walsh, R.N., Greenough, W.T. (Eds.): Environments as Therapy for Brain Dysfunction. Plenum Press, New York 1976; pp.132–170.

PETIT, T.L., ALFANO, D.P.: Differential rearing following developmental lead exposure: Effects on brain and behavior. Pharmacol. Biochem. & Behav. (in press).

PLATT, J.R.: Strong inference. Science *146*, 347–353, 1964.

POON, L.W.: A systems approach for the assessment and treatment of memory problems. In: Ferguson, J., Taylor, C.B. (Eds.): A Comprehensive Handbook of Behavioral Medicine. Spectrum Publications, Jamaica/New York (in press).

PREMACK, A.J., PREMACK, D.: Teaching language to an ape. Scientific Am. *227*, 92–99, 1972.

RAAIJMAKERS, W.: Brain cholinesterase activity. Doctoral thesis, University of Nijmegen, Netherlands 1978.

ROSE, F.C., SYMONDS, C.P.: Persistent memory defect following encephalitis. Brain *94*, 661–668, 1971.

ROSENBLUM, L.A.: Kinship interaction patterns in pigtail and bonnet macaques. Proc. 3rd Internat. Congr. Primatol., Zurich *3*, 79–84, 1971.

ROSENZWEIG, M.R., BENNETT, E.L.: Effects of differential environments on brain weights and enzyme activities in gerbils, rats, and mice. Dev. Psychobiol. *2*, 87–95, 1969.

ROSENZWEIG, M.R., BENNETT, E.L.: Cerebral changes in rats exposed individually to an enriched environment. J. Comp. Physiol. Psychol. *80*, 304–313, 1972.

ROSENZWEIG, M.R., BENNETT, E.L.: Enriched environments: Facts, factors, and fantasies. In: Petrinovich, L., McGaugh, J.L. (Eds.): Knowing, Thinking, and Believing. Plenum Press, New York 1976; pp.179–212.

ROSENZWEIG, M.R., BENNETT, E.L.: Effects of environmental enrichment or impoverishment on learning and on brain values in rodents. In: Oliverio, A. (Ed.): Genetics, Environment, and Intelligence. Elsevier/North-Holland, Amsterdam 1977; pp.163–195.

ROSENZWEIG, M.R., BENNETT, E.L.: Experiential influences on brain anatomy and brain chemistry in rodents. In: Gottlieb, G. (Ed.): Studies on the Development of Behavior and the Nervous System, vol.4, Early Influences. Academic Press, New York 1978; pp.289-327.

ROSENZWEIG, M.R., BENNETT, E.L.: How plastic is the nervous system? In: Ferguson, J., Taylor, C.B. (Eds.): A Comprehensive Handbook of Behavioral Medicine. Spectrum Publications, Jamaica/New York (in press).

ROSENZWEIG, M.R., BENNETT, E.L., DIAMOND, M.C.: Brain changes in response to experience. Scientific Am. *226* (2), 22-29, 1972a.

ROSENZWEIG, M.R., BENNETT, E.L., DIAMOND, M.C.: Chemical and anatomical plasticity of brain: Replications and extensions, 1970. In: Gaito, J. (Ed.): Macromolecules and Behavior, 2nd ed. Appleton-Century-Crofts, New York 1972b; pp.205-277.

ROSENZWEIG, M.R., BENNETT, E.L., HEBERT, M., MORIMOTO, H.: Social grouping cannot account for cerebral effects of enriched environments. Brain Res. *158,* 563-576, 1978.

ROSENZWEIG, M.R., BENNETT, E.L., MORIMOTO, H., HEBERT, M.: Lesions in occipital cortex of rat lead to secondary loss of cells in other cortical regions. Soc.Neurosci.Abstrs. *4,* 478, 1978.

ROSENZWEIG, M.R., KRECH, D., BENNETT, E.L.: Heredity, environment, brain biochemistry, and learning. In: Current Trends in Psychological Theory. University of Pittsburgh Press, Pittsburgh 1961; pp.87-110.

ROSENZWEIG, M.R., KRECH, D., BENNETT, E.L., DIAMOND, M.C.: Effects of environmental complexity and training on brain chemistry and anatomy: A replication and extension. J.Comp.Physiol.Psychol. *55,* 429-437, 1962.

ROSENZWEIG, M.R., SHERMAN, P.W., BENNETT, E.L.: Effects of differential environments on brain development in Belding's ground squirrels. In preparation.

ROZIN, P.: The psychobiological approach to human memory. In: Rosenzweig, M.R., Bennett, E.L. (Eds.): Neural Mechanisms of Learning and Memory. MIT Press, Cambridge 1976; pp.3-48.

RUMBAUGH, D.M., VON GLASERFELD, E., WARNER, H., PISANI, P., GILL, T., BROWN, J., BELL, C.: A computer-controlled language training system for investigating the language skills of young apes. Behav.Res.Methods & Instrumentation *5,* 382-392, 1973.

SAGAN, C.: The Dragons of Eden. Random House, New York 1977; p.263.

SANDERS, M.D., WARRINGTON, E.K., MARSHALL, J., WEISKRANTZ, L.: ‹Blindsight› : Vision in a field defect. Lancet *20,* 707-708, 1974.

SCHWARTZ, S.: Effect of neonatal cortical lesions and early environmental factors on adult rat behavior. J.Comp.Physiol.Psychol. *57,* 72-77, 1964.

SCOVILLE, W.B., MILNER, B.: Loss of recent memory after bilateral hippocampal lesions. J.Neurol., Neurosurg., & Psychiatry *20,* 11-21, 1957.

SIGNORET, J.-L., LHERMITTE, F.: The amnesic syndromes and the encoding process. In: Rosenzweig, M.R., Bennett, E.L. (Eds.): Neural Mechanisms of Learning and Memory. MIT Press, Cambridge 1976; pp.67-75.

170

SINGER, P.: Animal Liberation: New Ethics for Our Treatment of Animals. Random House, New York 1975; p.301.

STARR, A., PHILLIPS, L.: Verbal and motor memory in the amnestic syndrome. Neuropsychologia 8, 75–88, 1970.

STEIN, D.G., BUTTERS, N., ROSEN, J.: A comparison of two and four-stage ablations of sulcus principalis on recovery of spatial performance in the rhesus monkey. Neuropsychologia 15, 179–182, 1977.

STEIN, D.G., ROSEN, J.J., BUTTERS, N. (Eds.): Plasticity and Recovery of Function in the Central Nervous System. Academic Press, New York 1974; p.516.

STEWART, J.W., ADES, H.W.: The time factor in reintegration of a learned habit after temporal lobe lesions in the monkey *(Macaca mulatta)*. J. Comp.Physiol.Psychol. 44, 479–486, 1951.

UYLINGS, H.B.M., KUYPERS, K., VELTMAN, W.A.M.: Environmental influences on the neocortex in later life. In: Corner, M.A. (Ed.): Maturation of the Nervous System. Progress in Brain Research, vol.48. Elsevier/North-Holland Biomedical Press, Amsterdam 1978; pp.261–272.

VICTOR, M., ADAMS, R.D., COLLINS, G.H.: The Wernicke-Korsakoff Syndrome. F.A.Davis, Philadelphia 1971; p.206.

WALSH, R.N., BUDTZ-OLSEN, O.E., PENNY, J.E., CUMMINS, R.A.: The effects of environmental complexity on the histology of the rat hippocampus. J.Comp.Neurol. 137, 361–365, 1969.

WALSH, R.N., CUMMINS, R.A.: Neural responses to therapeutic sensory environments. In: Walsh, R.N., Greenough, W.T. (Eds.): Environments as Therapy for Brain Dysfunction. Plenum Press, New York 1976; pp.171–200.

WALSH, R.N., GREENOUGH, W.T. (Eds.): Environments as Therapy for Brain Dysfunction. Plenum Press, New York 1976; p.376.

WARD, A.A., Jr., KENNARD, M.A.: Effect of cholinergic drugs on recovery of function following lesions of the central nervous system in monkeys. Yale J.Biol.Med. 15, 189–229, 1942.

WARREN, J.M., KOLB, B.: Generalizations in neuropsychology. In: Finger, S. (Ed.): Recovery from Brain Damage. Plenum Press, New York 1978; pp.35–48.

WARRINGTON, E.K., WEISKRANTZ, L.: A study of learning and retention in amnesic patients. Neuropsychologia 6, 283–291, 1968.

WASHBURN, S.L.: Human behavior and the behavior of other animals. Am. Psychologist 33, 405–418, 1978.

WEISKRANTZ, L.: Trying to bridge some neuropsychological gaps between monkey and man. Brit.J.Psychol. 68, 431–445, 1977.

WEISKRANTZ, L., WARRINGTON, E.K.: The problem of the amnesic syndrome in man and animals. In: Isaacson, R.L., Pribram, K.H. (Eds.): The Hippocampus, vol.2. Plenum Press, New York 1975.

WEISKRANTZ, L., WARRINGTON, E.K., SANDERS, M.D., MARSHALL, J.: Visual capacity in the hemianopic field following a restricted occipital ablation. Brain 97, 709–728, 1974.

WELLS, A.M., GEIST, C.R., ZIMMERMANN, R.R.: Influence of environmental and nutritional factors on problem solving in the rat. Percep.Mot. Skills *35*, 235–244, 1972.

WEST, R.W., GREENOUGH, W.T.: Effect of environmental complexity on cortical synapses of rats: Preliminary results. Behav.Biol. *7*, 279–284, 1972.

WILL, B.E.: Methods for promoting functional recovery following brain damage. In: Berenberg, S.R. (Ed.): Brain, Fetal and Infant: Current Research on Normal and Abnormal Development. Martinus Nijhoff, Amsterdam 1978; pp.330–344.

WILL, B.E., ROSENZWEIG, M.R.: Effets de l'environnement sur la récupération fonctionnelle après lésions cérébrales chez des rats adultes. Biol. Behav. *1*, 5–16, 1976.

WILL, B.E., ROSENZWEIG, M.R., BENNETT, E.L.: Effects of differential environments on recovery from neonatal brain lesions, measured by problem-solving scores. Physiol.Behav. *16*, 603–611, 1976.

WILL, B.E., ROSENZWEIG, M.R., BENNETT, E.L., HEBERT, M., MORIMOTO, H.: Relatively brief environmental enrichment aids recovery of learning capacity and alters brain measures after postweaning brain lesions in rats. J.Comp.Physiol.Psychol. *91*, 33–50, 1977.

WILL, B.E., SUTTER, A.R., OFFERLIN, M.R.: Effets de la méthamphétamine et d'un environnement complexe sur la récuperation comportementale après atteinte cérébrale. Psychopharmacologia *51*, 273–277, 1977.

WOODWORTH, R.S.: Shepard Ivory Franz. Am.J.Psychol. *46*, 151–152, 1934.

ZIHL, J., VON CRAMON, D.: Restitution of visual function in patients with cerebral blindness. J.Neurol., Neurosurg., & Psychiatry *42*, 312–322, 1979.

Acknowledgments

The research of the author and his colleagues reported here was partially supported by a grant from the Easter Seal Foundation and by ADAMHA Grant R01-MH26704, and it received support from the Division of Biomedical and Environment Research of the U.S. Energy Research and Development Administration through the Laboratory of Chemical Biodynamics, Lawrence Berkeley Laboratory.

Preparation of this review benefitted from discussions with my colleagues Edward L.Bennett and Frank A.Beach, and I am happy to acknowledge their aid.

Brain control of movement: Possible mechanisms of functional reorganization

Edward V. Evarts

This report will present some highlights of neurophysiological studies relevant to the functional reorganization which occurs following damage to the motor cortex, the basal ganglia, or the cerebellum. As shown in Fig. 1, these three structures are interconnected, with cerebellum and basal ganglia projecting to motor cortex via thalamus. The input to motor cortex from thalamus has a critical role in generating volitional movement. A second major input reaches the motor cortex

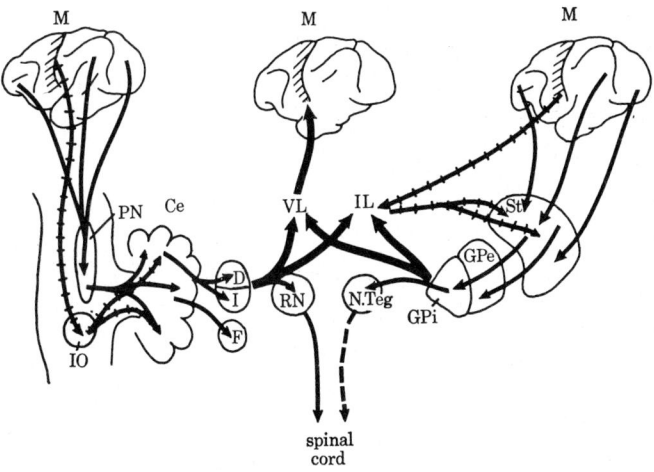

Figure 1. Cerebral connections of the cerebellum and basal ganglia. Ce: cerebellar cortex; D: dentate nucleus; F: fastigial nucleus; GPe: globus pallidus, external segment; GPi: globus pallidus, internal segment; I: nucleus interpositus; IL: intralaminar nuclei of the thalamus; IO: inferior olive; M: motor cortex; N. Teg: tegmental nuclei; PN: pontine nuclei; RN: red nucleus; St: striatum; VL: ventrolateral nucleus of the thalamus. (Reprinted from KEMP and POWELL, 1971.)

from the postcentral somatosensory area via a corticocortical projection which provides short-latency somatosensory feedback underlying servo-control of motor cortex output. During active movement these two inputs – thalamocortical and corticocortical – constantly interact to regulate the motor cortex signals which descend to spinal cord to control motoneuronal discharge.

The basal ganglia receive inputs from many cortical areas, including both sensorimotor and associative regions of cerebral cortex, and disturbances of the outputs from basal ganglia back to motor cortex (e.g., in parkinsonism) are particularly disruptive in relation to internally generated movements. Experiments in subhuman primates (HORE, MEYER-LOHMANN & BROOKS [8]) have shown that restoration of function following basal ganglia damage can sometimes be brought about by providing external sensory guidance in place of the subject's own internal guidance during movement.

The phylogenetically newer divisions of cerebellum, like the basal ganglia, receive strong inputs from the sensory and motor areas of the cerebral cortex. But the prefrontal and temporal areas of cerebral cortex, which project strongly to basal ganglia, fail to project to cerebellum. A current notion (cf. MILES & EVARTS [11]) as to cerebellar function holds that the Purkinje cells of the cerebellar cortex are summing points receiving both efference copy (from central sources) and afferent feedback (from the periphery). Purkinje cell outputs may provide «error signals» which are important in continuous regulation of movement.

Knowledge as to how motor cortex neurons participate in volitional movement is now being provided by studies of brain cell activity recorded in the monkey. Fig. 2 illustrates the technical procedures involved in such recording: a hollow cylinder is attached to the skull of the monkey, and a microelectrode is lowered through the cylinder into the underlying brain. When the microelectrode is sufficiently close to a given nerve cell, it will pick up a larger electrical signal from this nerve cell than from other nerve cells, and many successive observations on the different sorts of single nerve cells within a given brain area allow the neurophysiologist to infer the overall behavior of cells in that part of the brain.

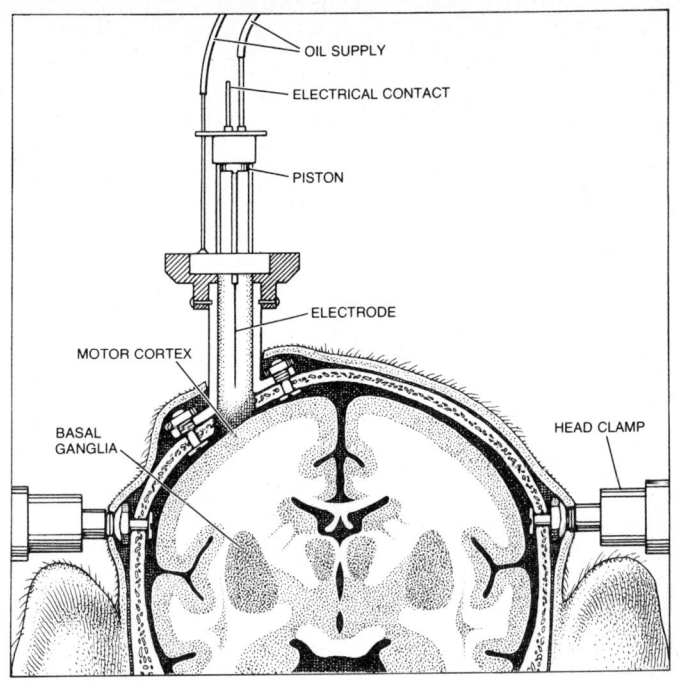

Figure 2. Microelectrode assembly consists of a fine platinum-iridium wire attached to a hydraulically actuated piston. A stainless steel cylinder permanently attached to the monkey's skull provides access to the brain. The bolts on the sides of the skull are also permanently implanted. They are attached to clamps during the experiment to prevent head movement. After the electrode assembly is bolted to the cylinder, the electrode is lowered by pumping oil into the inlet on the right and raised by pumping oil into the inlet on the left. (Reprinted from EVARTS, 1973.)

It is well known that motor cortex lesions are particularly disruptive with respect to precise movements of the extremities, and the experiments now to be described have provided information concerning motor cortex activity in relation to such movements. Fig. 3 illustrates the experimental paradigm: monkeys were rewarded for maintaining alignment between a track lamp and a target lamp, and learned to make precise arm movements to maintain this alignment. A pronation-supination arm movement of 1.5° moved the track lamp

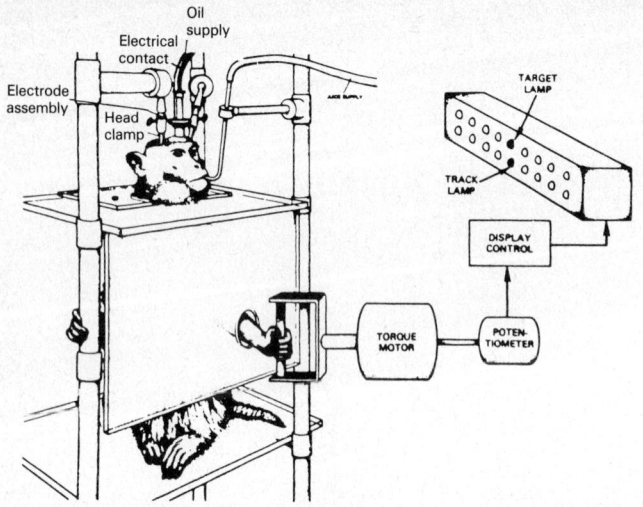

Figure 3. Visual pursuit tracking paradigm. The movements of the handle grasped by the monkey changed a potentiometer output which controlled the position of the track lamp. Displacements of the hand could be produced by the torque motor. The monkey was required to maintain alignment between track lamp and target lamp. (Reprinted from EVARTS, 1979.)

from one position to the next. Using such a paradigm (FROMM & EVARTS [6, 7], EVARTS & FROMM [4, 5]), the relation of motor cortex neuron discharge to precisely controlled visually triggered movements was studied in monkeys maintaining alignment of the lamps in the two rows. Also shown in Fig. 3 is a torque motor. Changes in the current through the torque motor deflected the handle grasped by the monkey and thereby delivered afferent inputs to the hand. Motor cortex responses to such stimuli (delivered during volitional movement) provided information as to the interaction between central programs and afferent feedback to motor cortex from limb receptors.

An example of motor cortex neuron activity in association with precisely controlled movement is given in Fig. 4, illustrating the discharges of a motor cortex neuron during small pronation and supination movements. At the upper left of

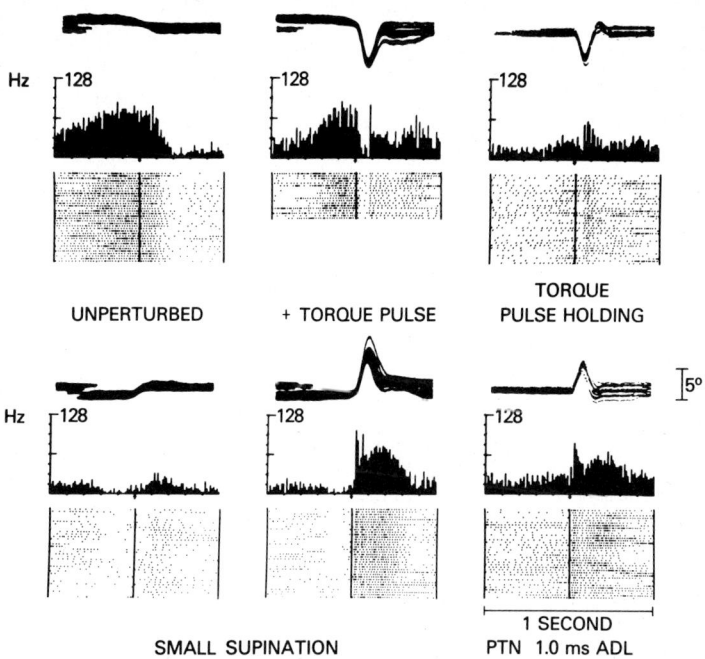

SMALL PRONATION

Hz

UNPERTURBED   + TORQUE PULSE   TORQUE PULSE HOLDING

Hz

SMALL SUPINATION

1 SECOND
PTN 1.0 ms ADL

Figure 4. Three sorts of displays are shown: (1) superimposed position traces, (2) histograms of unit discharge, and (3) rasters of unit discharge. Attention is directed to several points: (1) the inhibitory effect of the torque pulse is greater when it is delivered during a small pronation (top row, center, marked «+ torque») than when it is delivered during holding (top row, right, marked «torque pulse holding»). (2) There is a corresponding accentuation of the excitatory effects of the supinating torque pulse when this is delivered during small movement (bottom, center, marked «+ torque») as compared to holding (bottom, right, marked «torque pulse holding»). For further details, see text. (Reprinted from EVARTS and FROMM, 1978.)

Fig. 4 are traces corresponding to output of a position transducer coupled to the handle grasped by the monkey. The small downward deflection at the center of the position trace corresponds to a pronation movement of about 1°. Beneath the position traces are two different sorts of displays which depict the discharges of a motor cortex pyramidal tract neuron (PTN) which was reciprocally related to small pronation and supination movements. One of these displays (with ordinate marked 128 Hz) is a histogram showing discharge frequencies before, during, and after the small pronation movement. Below the bar histogram is what is referred to as a «raster,» where each *row* in the raster corresponds to one trial in which the monkey made a small pronation movement and where each *dot* in a given row of the raster corresponds to one impulse of the PTN. It is apparent that this particular neuron shows intense discharge with a small pronation movement (upper left). An opposite pattern of neuronal discharge occurs with a small supination movement (lower left), where supination is indicated by an upward deflection in the position trace: whereas the neuron became intensely active with a small pronation movement (upper left), it fell silent with a small supination movement (lower left). At the right in Fig. 4 are shown the responses of this same neuron to a *passive* pronation or supination occurring as a result of a motor-produced handle movement rather than as a result of the volitional movement of the monkey. It may be seen that this neuron was excited by a passive displacement which supinated (lower right) and was inhibited by a passive displacement which pronated (upper right). Note that there was *increased* activity of the neuron in response to an externally produced passive supination whereas there was *decreased* activity in association with a volitional active supination movement (compare active supination at lower left with passive supination at lower right). The center sections of Fig. 4 show how afferent feedback resulting from somesthetic inputs delivered to the hand interacts with the centrally programmed PTN discharge underlying voluntary movement. Afferent inputs produced by an external displacement which *opposes* the movement with which a given PTN discharges will *enhance* the discharge of the neuron, whereas afferent inputs produced by a displacement which *assists* the movement with which the neuron discharges will *diminish* neuronal discharge. Thus, for the PTN in Fig. 4, a passive external supination displacement *opposes* the active voluntary pronation movement with which the PTN discharges, and this external opposition excites intense

PTN activity (Fig. 4, lower center). The results shown in Fig. 4 are consistent with Phillips' [13] hypothesis that PTNs are summing points in a transcortical loop. For such a servo loop, realization of the action resulting from discharge of the PTNs should tend to reduce (i.e., to inhibit) discharge, whereas failure of realization should tend to increase (i.e., to excite) discharge. This is merely a restatement of the Phillips' hypothesis as to the effect of «match» and «mismatch» on PTN discharge. A familiar circuit exhibiting such negative feedback is the loop involving muscle receptors and alpha-motoneurons (α-MNs). Within this loop, the consequences of α-MN discharge (decreased muscle length and/or increased muscle tension) feedback onto the α-MN so as to reduce α-MN discharge:

$\downarrow$ muscle length $\rightarrow \downarrow$ muscle spindle discharge $\rightarrow \downarrow$ α-MN discharge

$\uparrow$ muscle tension $\rightarrow \uparrow$ Golgi tendon organ discharge $\rightarrow \downarrow$ α-MN discharge

The motor cortex PTN shown in Fig. 4 appears to be in a loop analogous to the one impinging on spinal cord α-MNs, a loop carrying information such that externally induced (i.e., passive) movement corresponding to the active movement called for by the PTN inhibits the PTN's discharge. By analogy with the model of negative feedback presented for the α-MN, an external «assist» which helps to realize the movement «commanded» by the discharge of the PTN will inhibit its discharge, whereas application of a force which opposes this movement will excite the PTN.

The motor cortex neurons with this precise input-output coupling in relation to pronation-supination are concentrated in a rather small cortical region which we can refer to as the cortical focus for control of supination-pronation movements. But the margins of this focus are not abrupt, and even beyond the «focal representation» for a particular movement there is a gradually diminishing fringe of neurons which can «take over» motor control when the focal area is damaged.

Many of our current ideas as to the gradients of motor cortex foci have come from the work of Phillips and his colleagues, and out of this work has come the concept of the «corti-comotoneuronal colony,» a term referring to that collection of PTNs projecting monosynaptically to a single spinal cord motoneuron. The experiments (cf. PHILLIPS & PORTER [14]) revealing the extent of corticomotoneuronal colonies involv-ed intracellular recording of monosynaptic EPSPs from spinal cord motoneurons. After a given spinal cord motoneu-ron had been impaled with the intracellular microelectrode, the motor cortex surface was mapped with a roving focal anode delivering pulses which were near threshold for the di-rect excitation of PTN axons, so that the maps were subjected to little error due to physical spread of current or physiologi-cal spread of excitation. It was found that the projection area to a single motoneuron could be extensive (up to 13 mm square), that areas were sometimes multiple, and that a col-ony for a given motoneuron commonly overlapped with col-onies projecting to motoneurons of antagonistic as well as synergistic muscles. Fig. 5 provides a schematic representa-tion of overlapping corticomotoneuronal colonies. It is worth reiterating that the extent of such an individual colony is defined by monosynaptic projections from cerebral cortex to a *single motoneuron*. If one now thinks of the region oc-cupied by the *set of corticomotoneuronal colonies* projecting to *all the motoneurons* of a given muscle, one realizes that it is a region which is indeed extensive and which must of necessity overlap with regions projecting to motoneurons of other muscles – both agonists and antagonists.

The zone of overlap illustrated in Fig. 5 is one from which electrical stimulation evokes monosynaptic excitatory synap-tic potentials in motoneurons of two different muscles. It may be worthwhile to speculate as to the relationship between this overlap and the cortical focus for representation of a par-ticular movement. Let us imagine that the overlap zone in Fig. 5 is a focal area in which there is intermingling of PTNs con-trolling pronator and supinator motoneurons; such a focal area would receive sensory inputs which would modulate the motor cortex outputs (e.g., as in Fig. 4) controlling prona-tion-supination movements. Around the focus is a recruit-ment region containing neurons which participate in larger,

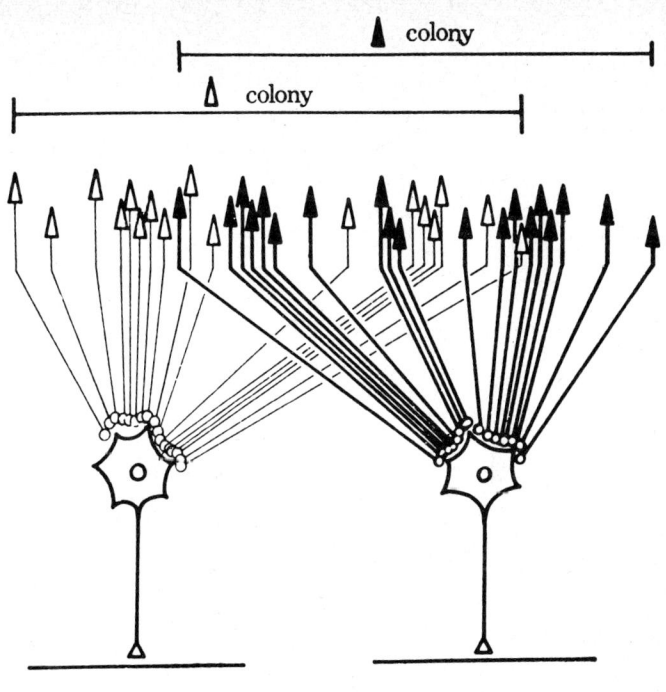

Figure 5. The filled triangles represent PTNs projecting monosynaptically to a single motoneuron, whereas the empty triangles represent PTNs projecting monosynaptically to a single motoneuron of a different muscle. Taken together, the filled triangles would constitute one corticomotoneuronal colony, while the empty triangles would constitute a second corticomotoneuronal colony. The two colonies overlap extensively. (Reprinted from PHIL-LIPS, 1969.)

more intense movements, but these fringe neurons do not receive such powerful sensory input in relation to the movement represented in the focus. It is postulated that recovery of function following damage to the focus for a particular movement may involve establishment of new connections from cortical areas which in the intact animal are in the recruitment fringe. It would seem that the recruitment fringe around the focus for a given movement may contain neurons within the focus for a *different* movement. Such fringe

181

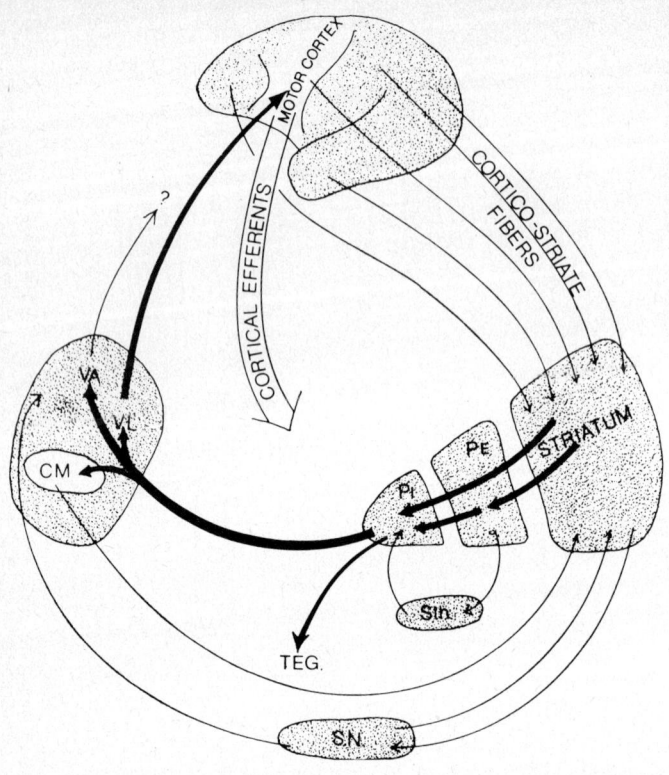

Figure 6. Summary of the major afferent, efferent, and intrinsic connections of the basal ganglia. The striatum (caudate-putamen) receives the majority of afferents to the basal ganglia. These come from three major sources: (1) the entire cerebral cortex, (2) the intralaminar nuclei of the thalamus, i.e., the center-median (CM), central lateral and parafascicular nuclei, and (3) the substantia nigra (SN). The striatum sends its output to the pallidum and the substantia nigra. The nigra gives rise to the well-known dopaminergic pathway to the striatum and also projects to the medial portions of the ventrolateral (VL) and ventroanterior (VA) nuclei of the thalamus. The internal division of the pallidum (P_i) gives rise to the major efferents from the basal ganglia, which terminate in the lateral portions of VL, VA, and CM and in the midbrain tegmentum (TEG). The projections from VA and VL to the prefrontal cortex provide a route whereby the basal ganglia can influence the motor and prefrontal cortex. Anatomically the basal ganglia are, in a manner of speaking, wired between the entire cortex on the one hand and the motor cortex on the other; i.e., they are «afferent» to the motor cortex. Direct descending influences from these nuclei do not extend below the midbrain. (Reprinted from DeLong, 1974.)

neurons have connections which allow them to assume control of new movements, given an adequate extension of their peripheral inputs and outputs within the spinal cord.

But while the discharge of motor cortex PTNs is regulated by afferent input during movement, its occurrence prior to movement is generated from within, and a major source of these internal inputs is the thalamus, which in turn receives its inputs from basal ganglia and cerebellum. Fig.6 illustrates some of the pathways involved in control of motor cortex by the basal ganglia. It may be seen that all regions of the cerebral cortex send fibers to the basal ganglia. The output of the basal ganglia via the thalamus is distributed preferentially to motor cortex. For what types of movement is integrity of basal ganglia particularly critical? Some intriguing observations relevant to this question have been provided by the work of HORE, MEYER-LOHMANN and BROOKS [8] in experiments showing that globus pallidus cooling disrupts learned arm movements of monkeys deprived of visual guidance, but that motor performance improves when visual guidance is made available. In the experiment of HORE et al., monkeys made extension and flexion movements of the elbow, and learned to do this with or without the assistance of visual feedback. The idea behind this experiment came from the long established clinical observation that visually guided movement may persist in patients with parkinsonism even when internally generated movements are greatly impaired. HORE et al. found that performance of movements in monkeys following globus pallidus cooling was much less impaired when vision provided feedback as compared to when it did not. When globus pallidus cooling had led to extreme motor disruption, dramatic improvement occurred when visual feedback provided the animal with information as to handle position. HORE et al. pointed out that the impaired ability to make alternating movements during contralateral globus pallidus cooling in the absence of vision is similar to the situation described in human patients.

The third brain region which will be discussed in this report will be the cerebellum, and its function will be considered in relation to its role in open-loop control systems with attention devoted specifically to the vestibulo-ocular reflex (VOR). ITO [9] has proposed that the cerebellar flocculus forms a side-loop regulating the relation between input and output in the open-loop VOR, and ROBINSON [15] has shown that lesions of vestibulo-cerebellum prevent the plasticity which underlies adaptive gain control of the VOR. Recovery following cerebellar lesions may involve behavioral substitution whereby slower closed-loop controls are used in place of fast open-loop controls for which cerebellar participation is vital. The pathway mediating the VOR involves the labyrinth, with the afferent fibers from the semicircular canals branching to the cerebellum and to the vestibular nuclei. It has been hypothesized that adaptive changes in the VOR take place by means of modifiable synapses in the cerebellum. Thus, a change in VOR gain has been thought to be due to changed Purkinje cell output passing from cerebellum to vestibular nuclei. The modification of cerebellar synapses is presumed to involve the action of climbing fibers reaching the cerebellum from the inferior olive. Studies of Purkinje cell discharge in the cerebellar flocculus in association with eye and head movement have shown that information concerning both eye velocity and head velocity reaches cerebellum, and that the Purkinje cell represents a summing point for these two classes of input. As a result of this summation, Purkinje cell discharge is modulated in relation to gaze velocity in space.

Adaptative gain control of the VOR was studied by MILES & FULLER [12] using monkeys fitted with spectacles which either enlarged or reduced the size of the retinal image. An enlarged retinal image called for an enhanced VOR, since with the enlarging spectacles a head movement of 5° would shift the retinal image by 10° and call for a 10° compensatory eye movement if the retinal image was to be stabilized. Use of spectacles which reduced the size of the retinal image called for a reduction of VOR gain. MILES & FULLER found a heightened VOR gain in animals who had worn the enlarging spectacles, whereas reduced VOR gain was found in animals who had worn reducing spectacles. The work of ROBINSON [15] has shown that the integrity of the cerebellum is essential for this adaptive plasticity of the VOR. ROBINSON found that normal cats wearing left-right reversing prisms exhibited VOR gain reductions of as much as 93%. This virtual elimination of VOR required about eight days; when the vestibulo-cerebellum was removed, the VOR gain rose to about one. The change in VOR gain resulting from reversing prisms was considered by ROBINSON to be an adaptive response designed to reduce image motion on the retina during head movements. It seemed clear that the vestibulo-cerebellum was necessary for this adaptive process, and ROBINSON proposed that detecting and repairing dysmetria was an important cerebellar function.

In conclusion, it has been proposed that the cerebellum may be of great importance in motor reorganizations which follow damage to other parts of the brain, since cerebellum may adaptively modify input-output relations and thereby compensate for changed information processing resulting from cerebral lesions. The basal ganglia appear to be especially critical in generating movements on the basis of internal mnemonic processes. Damage to the basal ganglia would seem to require shifts to other modes of motor control, especially to control via ongoing sensory inputs. The cerebral motor cortex is a final common pathway which receives thalamo-cortical inputs from basal ganglia and cerebellar systems. In addition to receiving these motor programs from cerebellum and basal ganglia, motor cortex receives cortico-cortical inputs which are of critical importance in the continuous guidance of precise limb movements on the basis of somesthetic inputs. The nature of motor cortex projection to spinal cord is such that surrounding each cortical focus for a particular movement is a fringe which in part controls the motoneurons involved in this movement but which may actually be in the focus for another movement. Recovery from restricted cortical lesions may involve a shift of control functions away from a damaged focus and into intact adjacent areas.

Bibliography

1 DeLong, M.R.: Motor functions of the basal ganglia: single-unit activity during movement. In: Schmitt, F.O., Worden, F.G. (Eds.): The Neurosciences. MIT Press, Cambridge, Mass. 1974; pp.319–325.

2 Evarts, E.V.: Brain mechanisms in movement. Sci.Amer. *229,* 96–103, 1973.

3 Evarts, E.V.: Brain mechanisms in voluntary movement. In: Neural Mechanisms on Behavior: The Texas Symposium (in press, 1979).

4 Evarts, E.V., Fromm, C.: Sensory responses in motor cortex neurons during precise motor control. Neurosci.Lttrs. *5,* 267–272, 1977.

5 Evarts, E.V., Fromm, C.: The pyramidal tract neuron as summing point in a closed-loop control system in the monkey. In: Desmedt, J.E. (Ed.): Cerebral Motor Control in Man: Long Loop Mechanisms, Progress in Clinical Neurophysiology, vol.4. Karger, Basel 1978; pp.56–69.

6 Fromm, C., Evarts, E.V.: Relation of motor cortex neurons to precisely controlled and ballistic movements. Neurosci.Lttrs. *5,* 259–265, 1977.

7 Fromm, C., Evarts, E.V.: Motor cortex responses to kinesthetic inputs during postural stability, precise fine movement and ballistic movement in the conscious monkey. In: Gordon, G. (Ed.): Active Touch. Pergamon Press, Oxford 1978; pp.105–117.

8 Hore, J., Meyer-Lohmann, J., Brooks, V.B.: Basal ganglia cooling disables learned arm movements of monkeys in the absence of visual guidance. Science *195,* 584–586, 1977.

9 Ito, M.: Neural design of the cerebellar motor control system. Brain Res. *40,* 81–84, 1972.

10 Kemp, J.M., Powell, T.P.S.: The connexions of the striatum and globus pallidus: synthesis and speculation. Phil.Trans.Royal Soc.B *262,* 441–457, 1971.

11 Miles, F.A., Evarts, E.V.: Concepts of motor organization. Ann.Rev. Psychol. *30,* 327–362, 1979.

12 Miles, F.A., Fuller, J.H.: Adaptive plasticity in the vestibulo-ocular responses of the rhesus monkey. Brain Res. *80,* 512–516, 1974.

13 Phillips, C.G.: Motor apparatus of the baboon's hand. Proc.Royal Soc. London B *173,* 141–174, 1969.

14 Phillips, C.G., Porter, R.: Corticospinal Neurones: Their Role in Movement. Academic Press, London 1977; p.450.

15 Robinson, D.A.: Adaptive gain control of vestibulo-ocular reflex by the cerebellum. J.Neurophysiol. *39,* 954–969, 1976.

Neuropharmacological aspects of brain plasticity

SIMÓN BRAILOWSKY

> Enfin, nul n'ignore les restaurations
> des fonctions psychiques, motrices
> et sensitives, même après les lesions
> graves des centres corticaux qui dé-
> terminent, par example, l'aphasie
> motrice, la surdité verbale, l'anes-
> thésie apoplectique, etc.
>
> S. RAMÓN Y CAJAL, 1911

I. Introduction

Clinicians concerned with the physical therapy and general rehabilitation of persons with incapacitating brain lesions rarely make use of drugs to alter the course of the disease, and in general, the pharmacological management of these patients is only symptomatic. For example, drugs that reduce spasticity following a stroke or the rigidity that accompanies Parkinson's disease merely provide temporary relief of symptoms or sequelae.

The majority of the ameliorative compounds originally came into use as a result of empirical observations, and with little or no understanding of the physiopathology involved. However, recent research has led to interesting hypotheses concerning the underlying mechanisms of action. In any case, the brain is considered so complex and delicate that any lesion sustained by this organ is usually and almost automatically given a grim prognosis.

These negative pronouncements – standard responses to central nervous system (CNS) lesions – reflect a certain resistance to the acceptance of facts that have been clearly demonstrated and/or an adherence to a mechanical type of dogmatism which can actually block the envisioning of favorable possibilities. A negative prognosis may be based more on the accompanying manifestations than on the pathological phenomena itself, since cause and effect are frequently confused at this level.

It is fitting to be humble with respect to the state of our knowledge concerning the brain. One should keep in mind that not all cerebral functions, especially those related at the molecular level to the degree of ocupation of receptors, have been or necessarily are detectable. In fact, the microphysiologist considers himself lucky to encounter a cell which is spontaneously discharging in the path of his microelectrode. The majority are in a «silent» state, firing only at the appropriate moment (LE GAL LA SALLE [36], SIEGEL & McGINTY [59]). Thus, a neuron is not required to be continously active for the function in which it is participating to persist: the existence of long-term memory and associated protein synthesis is an example. This is in keeping with the principle of economy in energy expenditure, and with what we might call physiological «minimal redundancy» in those functions which have become, through use, maximally automatized.

While the functions that we are aware of are far from being well-characterized, evidence from our daily lives indicates that they possess great adaptive potentiality. The range of nervous plasticity is not the same for every individual, nor is it constant throughout the life span of a single organism. Clearly, a capacity for change is not only manifested during early developmental stages, but rather is a life-long attribute of the nervous system. The adult organism continues to modify the performance of tasks depending on internal and external demands. Genetic expression undergoes a temporal evolution (e.g., certain proteins are only synthesized during a particular part of the life cycle), and there are also hereditary factors that determine an individual's specific response to the environment. Neuronal activity is regulated by synaptic input as well as by trophic factors that can influence membrane excitability and modify the expression of certain genetically coded patterns of activity (GUTMANN [25]).

Differences in nervous plasticity can be found at the regional level. Not all areas of the brain demonstrate the same responsiveness; for example, the cells of the cerebral cortex are anatomically and physiologically affected by the prenatal administration of growth hormone to a greater degree than those of the subcortical regions, indicating a difference in sensitivity (CLENDINNIN & EAYRS [8]).

The adaptability inherent in brain tissue is also evidenced after a lesion has been sustained. A pathological condition which remains unaltered for a long period of time is quite rare, and there generally are a number of functional changes that occur over the course of an illness. It could be said that a disease is not the same disease all the time and that the patient is not the same patient all the time; therefore, the clinician should not approach either one or the other with the same invariable orientation all the time.

As our knowledge of the CNS has advanced, we have extended the possibilities of favorably influencing those cases that require intervention. In medicine, pharmacology is one of the principal instruments for altering the course of a disease or preventing it altogether. The hypotheses that have been formulated in the past to account for functional recovery after CNS lesions have had to be modified under the influence of modern pharmacology. For example, the explanations of the underlying mechanisms of diaschisis (VON MONAKOW [66]) or denervation hypersensitivity, which has been better elucidated (GLICK [17]), have been greatly altered as experimental evidence for the possible existence of various neurotransmitters at the same synaptic terminal have been obtained (HÖKFELT et al. [29]) which would contradict the traditional concepts stated in Dale's Principle.

Pharmacology is the study of the effects of chemical substances on living matter. Included in the definition, however, is no mention of the factors which can modify this relationship.

Therefore, we shall begin this review of the neuropharmacological aspects of brain plasticity by briefly examining some of the factors pertaining to the drug itself, the subject, and the environment that can modify a drug's effect on cerebral tissue and plasticity, giving relevant examples from the literature whenever possible. In doing so, we seek to alert the clinician to some of the variables which can influence the results of clinical and experimental trials of new (or old) agents.

After giving this background which we hope will aid in the analysis of the following data, we shall review some of the research carried out on the use of drugs to facilitate nerve regeneration or functional recovery after CNS damage.

II. Factors that modify drug effects

The principal factors that determine the quantity and quality of drug effects are listed in Table I. It is important to bear in mind that our basic frame of reference is an altered nervous system.

1. Factors related to the drug

The majority of drugs act by combining with specific sites or macromolecules that normally are present in the cell. This interaction between drug and macromolecule depends on the physico-chemical properties of both elements, as well as on the conditions in which this interaction occurs. For a drug to produce a biological effect, it must possess a molecular structure that permits the establishment of bonds with the receptor. These bonds can be ionic, hydrogen (a strong dipole-dipole interaction), or effected through close-range electronic forces (London-van der Waals forces). This implies that apart from having a charge opposite to that of the receptor, the drug must possess a «molecular fitness» (stereo-selectivity or stereo-specificity) that is based on the three-dimensional structure (conformation) and molecular size (SASTRY [57]).

Little is yet known about the mechanism of action of pharmacological agents and, evidently, even less when this action takes place in a lesioned organism. However, the factors that determine the *access* of the drug to the receptor site are better characterized, and it is possible to correlate some of those

Table I. Factors that modify drug effects.

1. Factors related to the drug	molecular size and conformation degree of ionization lipid solubility	
2. Factors related to the subject	age gender physiological variables	body temperature sleep-waking cycles hormonal levels acid-base balance, etc.
	pathological states	CNS lesions (e.g., deafferentation, ischemia, trauma, etc.) immunological defects metabolic disorders infections, etc.
	genetic factors	variations in metabolism, sensitivity, immunological response, etc.
	psychological factors pre- and post-lesion exposure to drug	
3. Factors related to the environment	nutrition social variables medical facilities	setting lifestyle education, etc.
	pollution current styles	

which act at the level of the CNS with the theme that we are now developing.

In broad terms, the lower the molecular weight, the less ionized, and the more lipid soluble a drug is, the more rapidly will it pass through biological membranes and arrive at the site of action (e.g., the receptor). This rule is generally applicable to the absorption, distribution, biotransformation (metabolism), and elimination of any drug (see: GOLDSTEIN et al. [21]), and is valid in the CNS as well, with the addition of the factor of the so-called «blood-brain barrier» (OLDENDORF [44]).

It is know that a prime determinant in the distribution of a drug is the extent of the irrigation of the tissues (WILKINSON [73]). In the brain, a chemical substance has to cross not only the capillary wall (as in all other tissues with the exception of the placenta), but also the glial cell membrane which can surround up to 85% of the blood capillary (see: GOLDSTEIN et al. [21]).

This astrocytic membrane is by no means just one more barrier between the capillary endothelium and the neuron. There is a growing body of evidence testifying to the dynamic relationship that exists between glia and neurons:

a) Transference of protein material has been demonstrated between glia and neurons (GAINER et al. [16]).
b) «Typical synapses» between neurons and oligodendroglia have been found in the human cerebral cortex (TUSQUES et al. [63]).
c) The injection of sodium or lithium in glial cells evokes their depolarization, the discharge of adjacent neurons, and vascular pulsation (GROSSMAN & SEREGIN [24]).
d) Glial cells have been associated with recovery from experimentally induced demyelinating disease (HERNDON et al. [27]).
e) The administration of nerve growth factor (NGF) provokes hyperplasia and hypertrophy of the glial cells in the regenerating optic nerve of the newt (TURNER & GLAZE [62]).

It should be added that Dr. Rosenzweig's group (see Chapter 4) has demonstrated that glia also participate in the cerebral response to an enriched environment.

2. Factors related to the subject

Age. It is well known that younger individuals have an increased capacity or potentiallity for functional recovery after neural lesions (e.g. WEBER & STELZNER [69]). Drug action is age-dependent: the newborn and the old are more susceptible to many drugs, partially due to the immaturity or failure of detoxifying mechanisms (RICHEY & BENDER [51]). At the level of the CNS, a significant increase in the number of neuroglia has been reported in aging mice in the absence of any important alterations in the density of neuronal perikarya (STURROCK [61]). This suggests that the distribution of the drugs also may vary with age.

Gender. Although women have at times been called the «weaker sex,» recent experimental work has shown that female animals survive and recover more easily than males after pallidal lesions (LENARD et al. [37]). Nevertheless, they can display greater susceptibility to certain drugs, perhaps because of their generally smaller size, characteristic hormonal levels, or differences in the synaptic organization of the brain (GREENOUGH et al. [23]). These speculations are not entirely improbable since sex differences at the emotional and cognitive levels are already well known (e.g., GRAY & BUFFERY [22]).

Physiological variables. Body functions vary continuously according to environmental demands and internal states. For instance, during sleep there are alterations in electroencephalographic (EEG) rhythms, body temperature, muscle tone, respiration, hormonal levels, acid-base balance, etc. The response to a drug can be modified by these changes to a significant degree.

The influence of biological rhythms on drug action is illustrated in the effect of cyproheptadine on human volunteers (REINBERG & HALBERG [50]). It was reported that after the administration of the drug at 07:00, the effect lasted from 15 to 17 hours, while the same dose given at 19.00 was active for only 6 to 8 hours. The word «chronopharmacology» has been coined to define the new field of research that explores the relationship between drugs and biological rhythms.

The now-classic clinical report of the disappearence of abnormal movements of extrapyramidal origin (found, for example, in Parkinson's disease and Huntington's chorea) during sleep is relevant to this theme. ROWLAND [54] has found recovery of regulatory drinking in rats with lateral hypothalamic lesions predominantly at night.

Pathological states. The effects of drugs can dramatically change after an insult to the CNS has been received (e.g. ROTH & HARVEY [53]). Let us examine some of the possible events that may occur after a stroke or acute deafferentation. It is important to remember that there is a dynamic interplay between the structure of the brain and a pharmacological agent, so that the following phenomena can modify or themselves be modified by the effects of drugs:

a) Acute disequilibrium in the signal input-output ratio.
b) Metabolic disruption locally and in the homologous contralateral region.
c) Rebound of the non-affected antagonistic systems.
d) A «take-over» by priority (or hierarchical) systems.
e) Metabolic and functional alterations at the neighboring tissues, due in part to the accumulation of cellular lysis products (which may eventually become antigenic).
f) Denervation hypersensitivity of those areas innervated by the affected zone.
g) Increase in local inhibitory activity (possibly post-synaptically triggered) to compensate for hypersensitivity, etc.

Only some of these events have been clinically or experimentally demonstrated; the rest are hypothetical. Each of the above responses represents a possible level on which a drug might act or suggest a potential therapeutic approach.

Genetic factors. It is likely that the variability in the human response to drugs as well as in the capacity for functional recovery has a genetic basis. For example, BENNETT et al. [3] have shown strain differences among rats after exposure to enriched conditions, as measured by brain weight and cholinesterase activity. Moreover, the ageing process is influenced by hereditary factors, and both have been shown to be related to the degree of sensitivity to drugs. Another new field – that of pharmacogenetics – is developing (KALOW [32]).

Psychological factors. It has been demonstrated that pain perception alters with the time of day, mood, environment, expectations, hormonal levels, and other variables (KERR & CASEY [33], VON GRAFFENRIED [65]). In fact, we could say that all the factors listed in Table I, from age to current styles, are also applicable to pain.

The cognitive and emotional states of a patient before, during and after drug administration that are unrelated to the physico-chemical action of the drug itself and are responsible for the so-called «placebo effects», can sometimes make the difference between failure and success of the therapy.

In this regard, as Dr. BACH-Y-RITA will discuss (see Chapter 7), *motivation* becomes an important variable which may be manipulated pharmacologically, either directly or indirectly.

For example, we can enhance the drive of a spastic patient during physical therapy by administering a muscular relaxant which may increase and prolong his ability to perform the exercises. On other occasions, anti-depressants may be useful if his mood is dangerously low. However, it is important to bear in mind the possibility of fostering a psychological dependence on these compounds. The clinician must remain aware of this danger and be alert to any changes in the patient's attitude towards the drugs.

Pre- and post-lesion exposure to the drug. It has been reported that exposure to certain drugs prior to a lesion of the CNS can facilitate functional recovery (see: GOLDMAN & LEWIS [19]); however, the studies conducted on these findings have been basically descriptive up to now. They include quantification of the behavioral deficits (e.g., ROSNER [52], GOLDMAN & MENDELSON [20]), of post-lesion anatomical changes (e.g., LYNCH et al. [40], DEVOR & SCHNEIDER [12]), and of biochemical changes (HORN et al. [30], BERNSTEIN et al. [5]). From the pharmacological point of view, this phenomenon can be approached from at least two angles; exposure of the organism to a drug *before* the lesion is inflicted (which would imply a certain «learning» of the pharmacological effect), followed by a study of post-lesion responses (e.g., GLICK [17]); or, analysis of the effects of a drug in a lesioned organism that has never before been in contact with the agent, screening for possible qualitative changes («induced idiosyncrasy»). In some instances, the previous existence of a pathological condition is necessary for the «classic» pharmacological action to appear (e.g., conditions requiring anti-depressant drugs, anti-Parkinsonian agents, etc.).

3. Factors related to the environment

The significance of the context in which a drug is administered has received little attention up to now. When the environment and pharmacological action are mentioned together in textbooks, it is usually in reference to toxic effects (teratogenesis, intoxication, etc.), or to interactions with other substances (e.g., tobacco, alcohol). The characteristics of the historical and individual moment in which a drug is taken (aside from the subject's pathological condition) are only rarely taken into account. The relationship between biology and culture acquires special relevance here (see: RUFFIÉ [55], SAHLINS [56]), and developments in the fields of sociobiology and ethology promise to add new dimensions to the scientific study of man.

Rather than discussing the physico-chemical factors related to the environment that could modify pharmacological effects (e.g., temperature, humidity, barometric pressure, atmospheric radiation, etc.), we shall take this opportunity to briefly review some «non-classic» factors which, we believe, deserve more extensive study. It should be noted that the technological advances of our century have permitted the detection of certain environmental influences whose consequences we have steadily ignored, although we know of their presence. One example, the finding that exposure to electro-magnetic-fields tends to accelerate circadian rhythms in man (WEVER [72]), will suffice.

Nutrition. A history of malnutrition (which two-thirds of the world's children are estimated to have) automatically worsens the prognosis for recovery after a CNS lesion. These patients are more prone to infections and frequently exhibit associated pathology, aside from those alterations caused by malnutrition itself (see: PRESCOTT et al. [48]).

Social variables. The manner in which a patient lives can influence the process of therapy and influence recovery in several ways. For instance, he may be motivated either to return to work that he enjoys, or conversely, to hold pessimistic views about the future stemming from an aversion to his job.

In this case, motivation might be said to become a *socially determined variable.*

The effects of a medication can likewise be conditioned by the social milieu. An example drawn from the laboratory but which could easily be studied in clinical practice has been reported by SIEGEL [58]). He demonstrated that a change in environmental conditions alone, when administering morphine to rats, can cause the reappearance of an analgesic response in those animals that had already developed a tolerance to the narcotic. In other words, it is suggested that the setting (including, in the case of man, the *ritual)* which accompanies the dispensing of some and possibly all drugs can determine, at least quantitatively, the magnitude of the pharmacological effect.

The reactions of the people significant to the patient in matters of support, patience, and comprehension are also fundamental to the success of the treatment. Another laboratory finding which confirms the influence of social factors is that of an increased responsiveness to amphetamine in rats reared in isolation.

In these animals, isolation not only induces hyperactivity when they are exposed to an open-field test, but also, amphetamine selectively reduces this response (WEINSTOCK et al. [70]).

In many cases, education can provide a favorable framework for long-term treatment and is an example of an enriched environment for human beings. In some instances, however, education might block the successful development of a function, as in left-handed children whose parents pressure them to use the right hand «like everyone else».

Medical facilities. The accessibility of drugs is an important factor which is determined not only by price, sometimes excessive, but also by sheer geographic availability, such as the distance to the nearest hospital, physician or pharmacy. Needless to say, social security is far from being assured for everyone.

Pollution. The accumulation of potentially toxic materials in the atmosphere, water, and food has added a new and already voluminous chapter to toxicology. The physiological, immunological, and genetic consequences of pollution are not yet fully known, but will surely be widespread and on a large scale. Pesticides, lead, mercury, and food additives are a few of the many possible examples of substances that can modify drug action and which are now present in our environment (e.g., VESELL [64]).

Current styles. The sudden popularity of certain techniques, drugs, or surgical approaches, which is not related to their proven medical value, should also be mentioned as a factor which can interfere with the application of the scientific method.

Endorphines provide an excellent example of the dangers of *style*. These substances, present in mammalian brain, have been isolated and characterized very recently (see: COSTA & TRABUCCHI [10]). They produce pharmacological effects similar to morphine, such as analgesia and respiratory depression which are reversible upon the administration of the specific antagonist naloxone.

Obviously, the clinical implications of this discovery could be very important (e.g., these peptides might participate in phantom limb pain phenomena), but already – and at present with little basis – the endorphines have been related to diseases as different as schizophrenia and cancer.

The clinician must be aware of this «bandwagon» tendency and maintain a critical attitude when confronted with new and «sensational» experimental data.

III. Review of drugs used to influence recovery after CNS lesions

1. Cholinergic agents (Table II)

WOLF, in the 1940's, was one of the first scientists to attempt to facilitate recovery from brain lesions using drugs. At that time, the theory of chemical transmission at the nerve ending was still not widely accepted. He believed in the physiological importance of acetylcholine, the «vagusstoff» demonstrated by LOEWI in 1921, and tried to restore motor deficits in animals with apparently good results (WOLF [76]).

During World War II, members of Dr.Luria's group administered neostigmine (PERELMAN [45]) and later, galanthamine (PRAVDINA-VINARSKAYA & RUDAYA [47]), to patients suffering from brain wounds. Beneficial effects were reported following the use of these anticholinesterase agents. These experiments have not been repeated; some of the reasons for this lack of corroboration may be found in the pharmacological principles reviewed here. Neostigmine constains a highly ionized quaternary amine, which suggests that it has a poor capacity to move through the blood-brain barrier. This is not the case for physostigmine, another cholinesterase inhibitor which has a tertiary amine, a smaller degree of ionization, and consequently, the ability to produce greater central effects. For example, the intravenous administration of physostigmine to volunteers during slow-wave sleep can trigger the desynchronized phase (paradoxical or REM sleep) (SITARAM et al. [60]). The case of galanthamine is more complicated since it is a tertiary amine and the clinical effects that were reported are more impressive.

We feel that the «de-inhibitory» pharmacological treatment proposed by Luria's group should be investigated further, and if this work is still in progress, the results ought to be made more accessible. The therapeutic scheme which they advance consisting of rehabilitation based on a combination of appropriate exercises and drugs deserves serious consideration, and may provide a general framework for clinical research (LURIA et al. [39]).

Table II. Drugs used to influence recovery after CNS lesions. Cholinergic agents.

Drug	Species	Reported effects	Reference
Acetyl-B-methylcholine	Rat Cat	Accelerated recovery after sciatic nerve lesions.	WOLF, 1940
Neostigmine	Rat Cat	Accelerated recovery after sciatic nerve lesions.	WOLF, 1940
	Man	Aided recovery (using clinical criteria) from Bell's palsy and in one case of amyotrophic lateral sclerosis.	WOLF, 1940
	Man	Ameliorated paresis in patients with traumatic lesions.	PERELMAN, 1946
Carbamylcholine (C)	Monkey	Increased the rate of recovery of motor function after unilateral ablation of areas 4 & 6.	WARD & KENNARD, 1942
C+thiamine (T)	Monkey	Increased the rate of recovery of motor function after unilateral ablation of areas 4 & 6.	WARD & KENNARD, 1942
C+T+atropine	Monkey	Increased the rate of recovery of motor function after unilateral ablation of areas 4 & 6.	WARD & KENNARD, 1942
C+diphenyl-hydantoin	Monkey	Inhibited or prevented the enhanced recovery after the administration of C alone.	WATSON & KENNARD, 1945
Galanthamine	Man	Facilitated the re-education of wounded patients with disturbances of higher cortical functions.	PRAVDINA-VINARSKAYA & RUDAYA, 1959

The group of Dr. Margaret Kennard at Yale University also pioneered in this field (WARD & KENNARD [67], WATSON & KENNARD [68]). They administered cholinergic and anticholinergic agents as well as thiamine (vitamin B_1) to decorticated rhesus monkeys, obtaining an increase in the rate of recovery of motor function which, interestingly enough, could be blocked by the anticonvulsant compound diphenylhydantoin (DPH) (see Table VI).

2. *Stimulants* (Table III)

The Kennard group also used strychnine – a drug which has been shown to antagonize the effects of glycine, a putative inhibitory transmitter of spinal motor neurons – obtaining the same results in their animal model as with cholinergic agents.

This finding indicates a possible interaction between various transmitters, which could explain the clinical manifestations that are observed. The ability of this alkaloid to alter the effects on rat brain weight and cholinesterase activity found after exposure to an enriched environment has recently been tested, but yielded no results (BENNETT et al. [3]). It should be pointed out that these two studies are not easy to compare, since there are differences in the species and model employed.

Amphetamine and its derivatives have been the most investigated of the stimulant pharmacological agents in the context of recovery CNS lesions. As can be seen in Table III, these compounds appear to have beneficial effects in several animal models after central lesions were inflicted. However, it is necessary to remember that an increased level of arousal is required to obtain results in conditioning experiments.

Thus, the positive results could be due to this effect of amphetamine rather than to a more specific action on brain tissue.

The ages of the animals were very different in each of these experiments, further complicating the comparison of results.

Finally, Metrazole in sub-convulsant doses appears to exert no important effects (BENNETT et al. [3]).

Table III. Drugs used to influence recovery after CNS lesions. Stimulants.

Drug	Species	Reported effects	Reference
Strychnine	Monkey	Increased the rate of recovery of motor function after unilateral ablation of areas 4 & 6.	WATSON & KENNARD, 1945
	Rat	No change found in enriched environment effects.	BENNETT et al., 1973
D-amphetamine	Rat	Reversed the decremental effects of mammillothalamic tractotomy on avoidance behavior.	KRIECKHAUS, 1965
	Rat	Accelerated recovery of a visual conditioned response.	BRAUN et al., 1966
	Rat	Increased retention of an avoidance response after spaced occipital ablations.	COLE et al., 1967
	Rat	Enhanced enriched environment effects on brain weight and cholinesterase activity.	BENNETT et al., 1973
Methamphetamine	Rat	Enhanced enriched environment effects on brain weight and cholinesterase activity.	BENNETT et al., 1973
	Rat	No effects in animals with occipital cortical lesions (in contrast, beneficial effects of enriched environment were seen in these cases).	WILL et al., 1977
Metrazole	Rat	«Small positive effects» on brain weight and cholinesterase activity (after exposure to enriched environment).	BENNETT et al., 1973

Table IV. Drugs used to influence recovery after CNS lesions. Hypnotics and tranquilizers.

Drug	Species	Reported effects	Reference
Phenobarbital	Monkey	Slowed the rate of recovery after unilateral motor cortex lesions.	Watson & Kennard, 1945
	Rat	Decreased retention of an avoidance response after spaced occipital ablations.	Cole et al., 1967
	Rat	Decreased brain weight effects and increased enzymatic effects of enriched environment.	Bennett et al., 1973
Pentobarbital	Monkey	Promoted recovery after middle cerebral artery (MCA) occlusion.	Moseley et al., 1975
	Monkey	Protected against death due to MCA occlusion.	Michenfelder et al., 1976
Meprobamate	Monkey	Reduced the delay in conditioned responses which occurred after frontal lesions.	Weiskrantz et al., 1965
Haloperidol	Rat	Reduced the incidence of death and facilitated recovery after lateral hypothalamic lesions.	Hynes et al., 1975

3. Hypnotics and tranquilizers (Table IV)

The reports on the use of hypnotics and tranquilizers are somewhat conflicting: in general, barbiturates seem to impede recovery of function after central lesions but offer some protection against the acute effects of vascular occlusion.

Meprobamate, a minor tranquilizer with muscle relaxant properties, and haloperidol, a dopaminergic-receptor blocker which acts at the striatal, hypothalamic, and mesolimbic levels, have been reported to be effective in facilitating recovery after lesions, although once again, different animal models have been used.

4. Neuroregulators (Table V)

Neuroregulators are defined as those substances that can influence, directly or indirectly, communication between nerve cells (BARCHAS et al. [2]). All exert simultaneous complex actions at several levels of the CNS, making the interpretation of this data quite challenging.

HARVEY & SREBNIK [26] used L-thyroxine on rats suffering from compression of the spinal cord. They reported regeneration of the lesioned nerve fibers but offered no histological or electrophysiological evidence of this effect.

FERTIG et al. [14] administered the hormone triiodothyronine and corticotrophin (ACTH) to animals that had been sectioned at the telencephalic levels with damage to at least the internal capsule, corpus callosum, anterior commissure, and lateral olfactory striae. They reported beneficial effects.

BUSH et al. [7] also tested ACTH in animal with electrolytic lesions in the amygdala. The administration of the steroid one hour before shuttle-box testing resulted in the recovery of the deficits caused by the lesion. It would be interesting to know which neuroregulator(s) was/were affected by the lesion, since it is known that the amygdaloid complex contains at least a dozen of these substances.

The report of BERGER et al. [4] concerning nerve growth factor (NGF) is worth commenting on in some detail. NGF is

Table V. Drugs used to influence recovery after CNS lesions. Neuroregulators.

Drug	Species	Reported effects	Reference
L-thyroxine	Rat	Promoted axonal regeneration after spinal cord compression.	HARVEY & SREBNIK, 1967
Triiodothyronine	Rat	Enhanced axonal regeneration.	FERTIG et al., 1971
Corticotrophin (ACTH)	Rat	Interfered with normal scar formation.	FERTIG et al., 1971
	Rat	Facilitated recovery from shuttle-box avoidance deficits after amygdaloid lesions.	BUSH et al., 1973
Nerve growth factor (NGF)	Rat	Hastened recovery of feeding behavior after lateral hypothalamic lesions.	BERGER et al., 1973
Insulin	Rat	Facilitated recovery after dorsal hippocampal lesions.	DE CASTRO & BALAGURA, 1976
L-DOPA	Rat	Effected recovery from paraplegia induced by air injection into descending aorta.	POPOVIC et al., 1976

a protein, described by LEVI-MONTALCINI [38], that stimulates the growth and differentiation of peripheral sympathetic and sensory cells, as well as the sprouting and growth of regenerating noradrenergic neurons in the brain. BERGER and his colleagues found not only an acceleration of recovery from a lateral hypothalamic anorexic syndrome in rats, following an injection of NGF but also prevention of the re-initiation of the syndrome in the same animals which usually is caused by the application of 6-hydroxydopamine (a neurotoxin which destroys the dopaminergic terminals at the injection site). Thus, NGF appears to be a promising compound which should be tested in man after its central effects are better known.

It is possible that the positive results reported by DE CASTRO & BALAGURA [11] after the administration of insulin to rats with dorsal hippocampal lesions may have some relation to those produced by NGF, given the structural similarity of the two compounds (FRAZIER et al. [15]).

Finally, the effect of L-DOPA (L-3-(3,4 Dihydroxyphenyl)-L-alanine) reported by POPOVIC et al. (1976) appears to be peripheral, since low doses were employed (10 mg/kg) in the absence of decarboxylase inhibitors (normally, 95% of an L-DOPA dose is decarboxylated in the periphery).

5. *Other drugs* (Table VI)

We have grouped together in the last table a number of unrelated drugs which exert quite different effects. Diphenylhydantoin (DPH), a well-known anti-convulsant agent, produces no changes in monkeys with cortical lesions in areas 4 and 6 when administered alone. This compound is also included in Table II, as it modifies the effects of cholinergic agents. WATSON and KENNARD [68] found it to be «... capable of canceling the increased rate of motor recovery following medication with Doryl (carbamylcholine) alone» (p.228).

Several investigators have tested bacterial pyrogens (piromen, pyrogenal, pyronine) for their ability to modify the anatomical characteristics of scar tissue following lesions. They

Table VI. Drugs used to influence recovery after CNS lesions. Miscellaneous.

Drug	Species	Reported effects	Reference
Diphenyl-hydantoin	Monkey	No effects after motor cortex lesions.	WATSON & KENNARD, 1945
Bacterial pyrogens	Rat, cat monkey dog, man	Reduced scar formation after spinal cord sectioning.	WINDLE, 1955
«Neurocletin»	Rat	Induced sprouting after injection into muscles of normal animals.	HOFFMAN & SPRINGELL, 1951
Hyaluronidase and proteolytic enzymes	Rat	Promoted spinal cord regeneration after injection into transection site.	MATINIAN & ANDREASIAN, 1976
	Rat	Failed to alter scar formation in surgical central lesions.	KNOWLES & BERRY, 1978
α-Methyl-p-tyrosine (α-MPT)	Rat	Facilitated recovery after lateral hypothalamic lesions.	GLICK et al., 1972
p-Chlorophenyl-alanine (PCPA)	Rat	No effects after lateral hypothalamic lesions.	GLICK, 1974
Cyclophosphamide	Rat	Increased corticospinal axonal regeneration after spinal cord transection.	FERINGA et al., 1975
Azathioprine	Rat	No effects after spinal cord transection.	FERINGA et al., 1975
Morphine	Rat	Reduced the incidence of death and promoted recovery after hypothalamic lesions.	HYNES et al., 1975

sought to facilitate the passage of the surviving fibers in a proximo-distal direction through the tissue. Although this approach does not lack interest, the results were not conclusive and only touched upon one aspect of nerve plasticity: axonal regeneration.

«Neurocletin» (HOFFMAN & SPRINGELL [28]), a substance extracted from a combination of ox spinal cord and egg yolk, is an indication of the existence of thophic factors which originate in nervous tissue. The authors state: «… it is postulated that it (neurocletin) acts by disorganizing the cell membrane, and liquefying the axogel, resulting in outflow of axoplasm» (p. 424). Thus, it is a component of the axogel itself (possibly related to NGF?) which induces the sprouting.

The testing of proteolytic enzymes in rats with spinal lesions (see: MATINIAN & ANDREASIAN [41]) was carried out following the same rationale as that which prompted the use of bacterial pyrogens. It was reported that these substances promote spinal cord regeneration after transection by reducing scar tissue formation; however, these results could not be repeated in animals with central lesions (KNOWLES & BERRY [34]).

GLICK and his group at the Mount Sinai School of Medicine have approached the subject of the neuropharmacological aspects of brain plasticity from a quite original point of view. They have studied substances that interfere with the metabolism of putative monoaminergic neurotransmitters: α-methyl-p-tyrosine (an inhibitor of tyrosine hydroxylase and, consequently, of norepinephrine and dopamine synthesis), and p-chlorophenylalanine (an inhibitor of serotonin synthesis). Furthermore, they have evaluated the changes in pharmacological sensitivity to these compounds induced by CNS lesions (GLICK et al. [17, 18]). This strategy is a valuable one, in that it begins to make possible the description of changes that are induced by lesions (ADLER [1]) at the neurochemical level. For example: if we know that there exists a noradrenergic nuclear complex (locus coeruleus-subcoeruleus) at the level of the brainstem with diffusely projecting ascending and descending fibers, and furthermore, that at least in some regions, such as the cerebellum, the activation of these cells gives rise to inhibitory responses, we could deduce some of the effects which a lesion of the former area could produce – not only locally (e. g., in the cellular bodies and passing fibers), but also at a distance.

FERINGA et al. [13] have proposed the existence of allergic reactions caused by the liberation of antigenic substances which originate in lesioned axons. According to this supposition, the inhibition of the auto-immune response could facilitate the regeneration of the effected fibers. They have, in fact, reported an increase in corticospinal axonal regeneration after spinal cord transection using cyclophosphamide. However, one has to carefully weigh the advantages and disadvantages of a treatment which has deleterious effects on human beings.

HYNES et al. [31] administered haloperidol (see Table IV) or morphine to rats for six days prior to a bilateral lesion of the lateral region of the hypothalamus. They reported that this treatment promoted recovery and reduce the incidence of death; however, a replication of this experiment has not been published.

A number of the studies summarized above do not appear to be solidly based theoretically, and their inclusion in this chapter does not imply the agreement of this author with their approaches or conclusions.

IV. Conclusions

We believe that this work does not yet lend itself to conclusions of a practical nature which are directly pertinent to the long-term management of patients with cerebral lesions. Nevertheless, we shall venture some propositions of a theoretical nature whose application must be left to the clinician.

a) The CNS is not a static structure: it is modified by unfolding genetic patterns and undergoes changes which are both spontaneous and in response to environmental stimuli (including those attributable to lesions).

b) The functional unity of the CNS is based on its constitutive elements – fundamentally, neurons and glial cells. The CNS should be conceived of in these terms when attempts are made to explain the response to lesions or to the administration of drugs.

c) In the majority of cases, centrally acting pharmacological agents owe their effects to an interaction with specific sites in the cell, dependent on their physico-chemical properties and on the moment in which this interaction takes place (i.e., the state of the receptor).

d) In order to properly evaluate the response of the lesioned CNS to drugs, the principal factors capable of modifying pharmacological effects should be taken into account – those related to the drug, the subject, and the environment.

e) The response on the part of the lesioned organism to pharmacological substances can aid in the localization of the lesion and/or the site of action of the drug.

f) The effects of a CNS agent can change both quantitatively and qualitatively when administered to a lesioned organism.

g) The pharmacological treatment of patients with central lesions, when appropriate drugs become available, should be carried out within a framework of an integrated therapy that includes attention to the physical, motivational, and social aspects of the individual.

Acknowledgments

I am indebted to Drs. M.Shkurovich and J.L.Diaz for reading the manuscript and making valuable suggestions, and to Marcella Vogt for her expertise in the editing of this work.

Without the continuous encouragement of Dr. P.Bach-y-Rita, this chapter would not have been published.

Bibliography

1 ADLER, M.W.: General principles and problems related to the use of brain lesions. Psychopharmacol.Bull. *14,* 30–32, 1978.
2 BARCHAS, J.D., AKIL, H., ELLIOT, G.R., HOLMAN, R.B., WATSON, S.J.: Behavioral neurochemistry: neuroregulators and behavioral states. Science *200,* 964–973, 1978.

3 BENNETT, E.L., ROSENZWEIG, M.R., WU, S.Y.C.: Excitant and depressant drugs modulate effects of environment on brain weight and cholinesterase. Psychopharmacologia (Berl.) *33,* 309–328, 1973.

4 BERGER, B.D., WISE, C.D., STEIN, L.: Nerve growth factor: enhanced recovery of feeding after lateral hypothalamic damage. Science *180,* 506–508, 1973.

5 BERNSTEIN, J.J., WELLS, M.R., BERNSTEIN, M.E.: Spinal cord-regeneration: synaptic renewal and neurochemistry. In: Cotman, C.W. (Ed.): Neuronal Plasticity. Raven Press, New York 1978; pp.49–71.

6 BRAUN, J.J., MEYER, P.M., MEYER, D.R.: Sparing of a brightness habit in rats following visual decortication. J.Comp. & Physiol.Psychol. *61,* 79–82, 1966.

7 BUSH, D.F., LOVELY, R.H., PAGANO, R.R.: Injection of ACTH induces recovery from shuttle-box avoidance deficits in rats with amygdaloid lesions. J.Comp. & Physiol.Psychol. *83,* 168–172, 1973.

8 CLENDINNIN, B.G., EAYRS, J.T.: The anatomical and physiological effects of prenatally administered somatotropin on cerebral development in rats. J.Endocrinol. *22,* 183–193, 1961.

9 COLE, D.D., SULLINS, W.R., Jr., ISAAC, W.: Pharmacological modification of the effects of spaced occipital ablations. Psychopharmacologia (Berl.) *11,* 311–316, 1967.

10 COSTA, E., TRABUCCHI, M. (Eds.): The Endorphines. Adv.Biochem. Psychopharmacol., vol.18. Raven press, New York 1978; p.357.

11 DE CASTRO, J.M., BALAGURA, S.: Insulin pretreatment facilitates recovery after dorsal hippocampal lesions. Physiol.Behav. *16,* 517–520, 1976.

12 DEVOR, M., SCHNEIDER, G.E.: Neuroanatomical plasticity: the principle of conservation of total axonal arborization. In: Vital-Durand, F., Jeannerod, M. (Eds.): Aspects of Neural Plasticity. INSERM, Paris 1975; pp.191–201.

13 FERINGA, E.R., JOHNSON, R.D., WENDT, J.S.: Spinal cord regeneration in rats after immunosuppressive treatment. Theoretic considerations and histologic results. Arch.Neurol. (Chic.) *32,* 676–683, 1975.

14 FERTIG, A., KIERNAN, J.A., SEYAN, S.S.: Enhancement of axonal regeneration in the brain of the rat by corticotrophin and triiodothyronine. Exp.Neurol. *33,* 372–385, 1971.

15 FRAZIER, W.A., ANGELETTI, R.H., BRADSHAW, R.A.: Nerve growth factor and insulin. Science *176,* 482–488, 1972.

16 GAINER, H., TASAKI, I., LASEK, R.J.: Evidence for the glianeuron protein transfer hypothesis from intracellular perfusion studies of squid giant axons. J.Cell Biol. *74,* 524–530, 1977.

17 GLICK, S.D.: Changes in drug sensitivity and mechanisms of functional recovery following brain damage. In: Stein, D.G., Rosen, J.J., Butters, N. (Eds.): Plasticity and Recovery of Function in the Central Nervous System. Academic Press, New York 1974; pp.339–372.

18 GLICK, S.D., GREENSTEIN, S., ZIMMERBERG, B.: Facilitation of recovery by α-methyl-*p*-tyrosine after lateral hypothalmic damage. Science *177,* 534–535, 1972.

19 GOLDMAN, P.S., LEWIS, M.E.: Developmental biology of brain damage and experience. In: Cotman, C.W. (Ed.): Neuronal Plasticity. Raven Press, New York 1978; pp.291–310.

20 GOLDMAN, P.S., MENDELSON, M.J.: Salutary effects of early experience on deficits caused by lesions of frontal association cortex in developing rhesus monkeys. Exp.Neurol. 57, 588–602, 1977.

21 GOLDSTEIN, A., ARONOW, L., KALMAN, S.M.: Principles of Drug Action: The Basis of Pharmacology, 2nd ed. John Wiley & Sons, New York 1974; p.854.

22 GRAY, J., BUFFERY, A.: Sex differences in emotional and cognitive behavior in mammals including man: adaptive and neural bases. Acta psychol. (Amst.) 35, 89–111, 1971.

23 GREENOUGH, W.T., CARTER, C.S., STEERMAN, C., DE VOOGD, T.J.: Sex differences in dendritic patterns in hamster preoptic area. Brain Res. 126, 63–72, 1977.

24 GROSSMAN, R.G., SEREGIN, A.: Glial-neuron interaction demonstrated by the injection of Na^+ and Li^+ into cortical glia. Science 195, 196–198, 1977.

25 GUTMANN, E.: Neurotrophic relations. Ann.Rev.Physiol. 38, 177–216, 1976.

26 HARVEY, J.E., SREBNIK, H.H.: Locomotor activity and axon regeneration following spinal cord compression in rats treated with l-thyroxine. J.Neuropath. & Exper.Neurol. 26, 661–668, 1967.

27 HERNDON, R.M., PRICE, D.L., WEINER, L.P.: Regeneration of oligo-dendroglia during recovery from demyelinating disease. Science 195, 693–694, 1977.

28 HOFFMAN, H., SPRINGELL, P.H.: An attempt at the chemical identification of «neurocletin» (the substance evoking axon sprouting). Australian J.Exper.Biol. & M.Sci. 29, 417–424, 1951.

29 HÖKFELT, T., LJUNGDAHL, Å., ELDE, R.P., NILSSON, G., TERENIUS, L., GOLDSTEIN, M., STEINBUSCH, H., VERHOFSTAD, A.: Interdependence of neurotransmitters and systems – morphological basis. Abst.1313, p.508. Proc. 7th Inter.Congr.Pharmacol., Paris, July 16–21, 1978.

30 HORN, G., ROSE, S.P., BATESON, P.P.: Experience and plasticity in the central nervous system. Science 181, 506–514, 1973.

31 HYNES, M.D., ANDERSON, C.D., GIANUTSOS, G., LAL, H.: Effects of haloperidol, methyltyrosine and morphine on recovery from lesions of lateral hypothalamus. Pharmacol.Biochem.Behav. 3, 755–759, 1975.

32 KALOW, W.: Pharmacogenetics: Heredity and the Response to Drugs. W.B. Saunders, Philadelphia 1962.

33 KERR, F.W.L., CASEY, K.L. (Eds.): Pain. Neurosci.Res.Program Bull., vol.16. MIT Press, Cambridge 1978; p.207.

34 KNOWLES, J.F., BERRY, M.: Effect of enzyme treatment of central nervous system lesions in the rat. Exp.Neurol. 59, 450–454, 1978.

35 KRIECKHAUS, E.E.: Decrements in avoidance behavior following mammillothalamic tractotomy in rats and subsequent recovery with d-amphetamine. J.Comp. & Physiol.Psychol. 60, 31–35, 1965.

36 Le Gal la Salle, G.: Unitary responses in the amygdaloid complex following stimulation of various diencephalic structures. Brain Res. *118,* 475–478, 1976.

37 Lenard, L., Sarkisian, J., Szabo, I.: Sex-dependent survival of rats after bilateral pallidal lesions. Physiol.Behav. *15,* 389–397, 1975.

38 Levi-Montalcini, R.: The nerve growth factor: its role in growth, differentiation and function of the sympathetic adrenergic neuron. In: Corner, M.A., Swaab, D.F. (Eds.): Progress in Brain Research, vol.45. Elsevier, Amsterdam 1976; pp.235–258.

39 Luria, A.R., Naydin, V.L., Tsvetkova, L.S., Vinarskaya, E.N.: Restoration of higher cortical function following local brain damage. In: Vinken, P.J., Bruyn, G.W. (Eds.): Handbook of Clinical Neurology, vol.3. North-Holland, Amsterdam 1969; pp.368–433.

40 Lynch, G., Stanfield, B., Cotman, C.W.: Developmental differences in post-lesion axonal growth in the hippocampus. Brain Res. *59,* 155–168, 1973.

41 Matinian, L.A., Andreasian, A.S.: Enzyme Therapy in Organic Lesions of the Spinal Cord. Brain Information Service, Los Angeles University of California, 1976; p.156.

42 Michenfelder, J.D., Milde, J.H., Sundt, T.M., Jr.: Cerebral protection by barbiturate anesthesia. Arch.Neurol. (Chic.) *33,* 345–350, 1976.

43 Moseley, J.I., Laurent, J.P., Molinari, G.F.: Barbiturate – attenuation in the clinical course of pathologic lesions in a – primate stroke model. Neurology *25,* 870–874, 1975.

44 Oldendorf, W.H.: Blood-brain barrier permeability to drugs. Ann. Rev.Pharmacol. *14,* 239–248, 1974.

45 Perelman, L.B.: The pharmacological treatment of motor and sensory disorders after trauma to the central nervous system. Sov.Med. No.8–9, 1946.

46 Popovic, P., Popovic, V., Schaffer, R.: Recovery from experimental paraplegia after levodopa administration. Arch.Neurochir. *35,* 141–147, 1976.

47 Pravdina-Vinarskaya, E.N., Rudaya, G.B.: Re-education of the gnostical, praxical and speech functions, and disinhibition treatment with galanthaminum (Russian). Reports Acad.Pedagog.Sci. RSFSR No.5: 113–116, 1959.

48 Prescott, J.W., Read, M.S., Coursin, D.B. (Eds.): Brain Functions and Malnutrition: Neuropsychological Methods of Assessment. John Wiley and Sons, New York 1975; p.440.

49 Ramón y Cajal, S.: Histologie du Système Nerveux de l'Homme et des Vertébrés, Vol.II. Maloine, Paris 1911; pp.888–889.

50 Reinberg, A., Halberg, F.: Circadian Chronopharmacology. Ann. Rev.Pharmacol. *11,* 455–492, 1971.

51 Richey, D.P., Bender, A.D.: Pharmacokinetic consequences of aging. Ann.Rev.Pharmacol. *17,* 49–65, 1977.

52 Rosner, B.S.: Brain functions. Ann.Rev.Psychol. *21,* 555–594, 1970.

53 Roth, B.F., Harvey, J.A.: Altered response of cerebral respiration to

thiopental and potassium ions *in vitro* after septal lesions. J. Pharmacol. & Exper. Therap. *161*, 155–162, 1968.

54 ROWLAND, N.: Circadian rhythms and partial recovery of regulatory drinking in rats after lateral hypothalamic lesions. J. Comp. & Physiol. Psychol. *90*, 382–393, 1976.

55 RUFFIÉ, J.: De la Biologie à la Culture. Flammarion, Paris 1976; p. 594.

56 SAHLINS, M.: The Use and Abuse of Biology, 3rd ed. The University of Michigan Press, Ann Arbor 1977; p. 120.

57 SASTRY, B. V. R.: Stereoisomerism and drug action in the nervous system. Ann. Rev. Pharmacol. *13*, 253–267, 1973.

58 SIEGEL, S.: Morphine analgesic tolerance: its situation specificity supports a Pavlovian conditioning model. Science *193*, 323–325, 1976.

59 SIEGEL, J. M., McGINTY, D. J.: Brainstem neurons without spontaneous unit discharge. Science *193*, 240–242, 1976.

60 SITARAM, N., WYATT, R. J., DAWSON, S., GILLIN, J. C.: REM sleep induction by physostigmine infusion during sleep. Science *191*, 1281–1283, 1976.

61 STURROCK, R. R.: Quantitative and morphological changes in neurons and neuroglia in the indusium griseum of aging mice. J. Gerontol. *32*, 647–658, 1977.

62 TURNER, J. E., GLAZE, K. A.: Glial reaction to nerve growth factor in the regeneration optic nerve of the newt *(Triturus viridiscens)*. Exp. Neurol. *59*, 190–201, 1978.

63 TUSQUES, J., GEORGE, Y., ROCH, M.: Mise en évidence de synapses typiques entre neurones et oligodendrocytes dans l'écorce cérébrale humaine. C. R. Acad. Sci. (Paris) *283*, 1747–1749, 1976.

64 VESELL, E. S.: Genetic and environmental factors affecting drug disposition in man. Clin. Pharmacol. & Therap. *22*, 659–679, 1977.

65 VON GRAFFENRIED, B., ADLER, R., ABT, K., NÜESCH, E., SPIEGEL, R.: The influences of anxiety and pain sensitivity on experimental pain in man. Pain *4*, 253–263, 1978.

66 VON MONAKOW, C.: Die Localisation im Grosshirn und der Abbau der Funktion durch kortikale Herde. J. F. Bergmann, Wiesbaden 1914.

67 WARD, A. A., Jr., KENNARD, M. A.: Effect of cholinergic drugs on recovery of function following lesions of the central nervous system in monkeys. Yale J. Biol. & Med. *15*, 189–228, 1942.

68 WATSON, C. W., KENNARD, M. A.: The effect of anticonvulsant drugs on recovery of function following cerebral cortical lesions. J. Neurophysiol. *8*, 221–231, 1945.

69 WEBER, E. D., STELZNER, D. J.: Behavioral effects of spinal cord transection in the developing rat. Brain. Res. *125*, 241–255, 1977.

70 WEINSTOCK, M., SPEISER, Z., ASHKENAZI, R.: Changes in brain catecholamine turnover and receptor sensitivity induced by social deprivation in rats. Psychopharmacology *56*, 205–209, 1978.

71 WEISKRANTZ, L., GROSS, C. G., BALTZER, V.: The beneficial effects of meprobamate on delayed response performance in the frontal monkey. Quart. J. Exper. Psychol. *17*, 118–124, 1965.

72 WEVER, R.: Einfluss schwacher electromagnetischer Felder auf die circadiane Periodik des Menschen. Naturwissenschaften *55,* 29–32, 1968.

73 WILKINSON, G.R.: Pharmacokinetics of drug disposition: hemodynamic considerations. Ann.Rev.Pharmacol. *15,* 11–28, 1975.

74 WILL, B.E., SUTTER, A.R., OFFERLIN, M.R.: Effects of methamphetamine and enriched experience on behavioral recovery afterbrain damage. Psychopharmacology *51,* 273–277, 1977.

75 WINDLE, W.F.: Comments on regeneration in the human central nervous system. In: Windle, W.F. (Ed.): Regeneration in the Central Nervous System. Charles C.Thomas, Springfield, Ill. 1955; pp.265–271.

76 WOLF, A.: A method of shortening the duration of lower motor neurone paralysis by cholinergic facilitation. J.Nerv. & Ment.Dis. *92,* 614–622, 1940.

Appendix

Possible levels of pharmacological action at the synapse: A theoretical approach

S. BRAILOWSKY

Classical neuronal theory considers the nerve cell as the essential component for brain function; however, the total cell population of the central nervous system (CNS) is composed of neuroglia as well as neurons. The role of the glia has begun to be studied in detail and already has led to significant modifications in the classical theory (see WATSON, 1976). The neuron-glia system should be considered, then, as a functional entity which has, among other characteristics, plastic capacity.

Plasticity signifies change, which implies interaction. If the possibilities for interaction between various systems at the central level have phylogenetically increased, this advance has been due to an ever more rigorous control of the *milieu interieur,* which in turn is a response to the demands imposed by the surrounding environment. Thanks to the microtechniques currently available, the phenomenology of neuron-glia

215

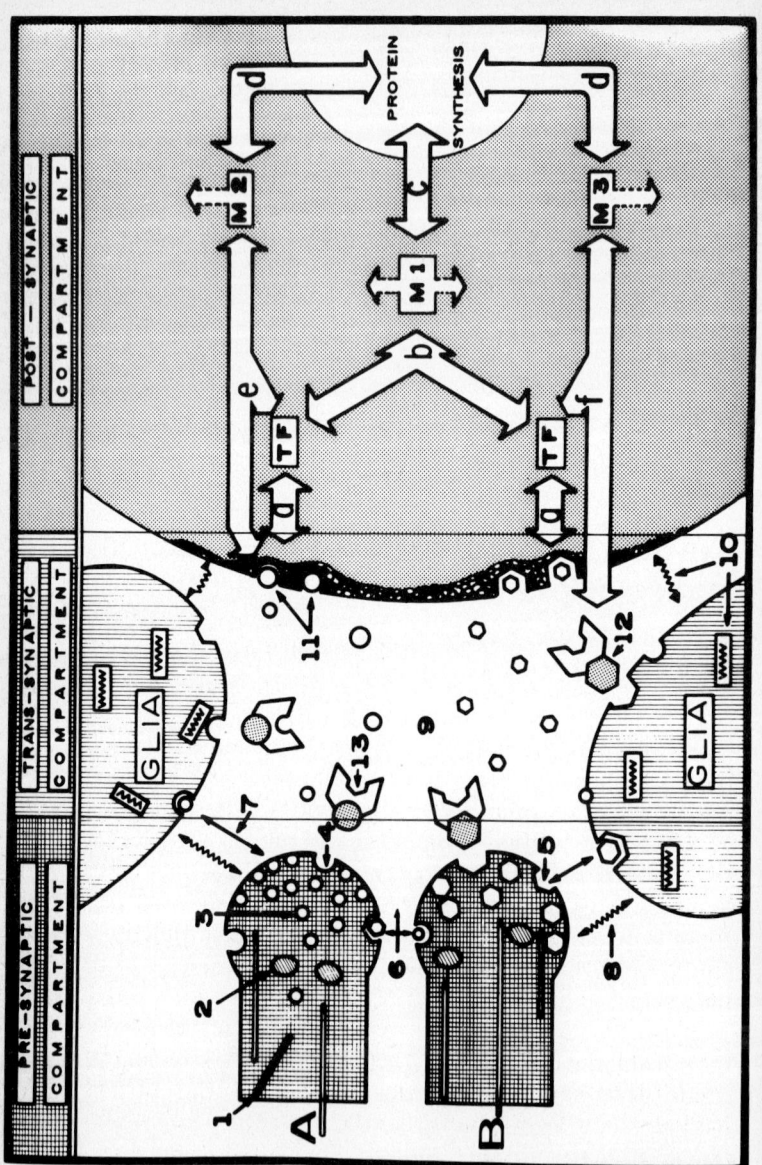

216

Figure 1. Model of a synapse.

I. Pre-synaptic compartment
   1. Axonal transport
   2. Synthesis of neuroregulator(s)
   3. Storage of neuroregulator(s)
   4. Release of neuroregulator(s)
   5. Presynaptic receptor and reuptake of neuroregulator(s)
   6. Presynaptic interaction mediated by neurotransmitter(s)
   7. Presynaptic terminal-glia interaction mediated by neurotransmitter(s)
   8. Presynaptic terminal-glia interaction mediated by peptide(s)
II. Trans-synaptic compartment
   9. Extracellular space
   10. Glia-neuron and glia-extracellular space interactions
III. Post-synaptic compartment
   11. Occupation of the receptor
       Postsynaptic events initiated by occupation of the receptor:
       a) Receptor-transducer interaction (TF: transduction factor)
       b) Transducer – first messenger (M1) interaction
       c) First messenger (M1) – cell nucleus interaction
       d) Protein synthesis – cytoplasmic messenger(s) (M2) interaction
       e) M2 messengers – TF and M2 messengers – membrane receptor interactions
       f) M3 messengers – TF and M3 messengers – protein synthesis of neuromodulator(s) interactions
   12. Postsynaptic release of specific neuromodulator(s)
   13. Postsynaptic release of neuromodulator(s) with multiple actions

---

interactions with the environment has begun to be described at the molecular level.

The model to be proposed in this addendum (Fig. 1) is a summary of, and has been constructed from, a series of fragmentary data on synaptic functioning, with the addition of several hypothetical steps or mechanisms that could be considered by the neuroscientist as suggestions for possible new lines of research. With this model, we hope to reveal the complexity of events involved in nervous transmission by breaking down the whole into parts, each one of which could constitute a site or level of pharmacological action.

In this scheme are included the basic synaptic components: presynaptic terminals of afferent neurons (A, B); the postsynaptic membrane and body of the effector neuron; glial cells; and the extracellular space. The synaptic zone has been arbitrarily subdivided into three (pre-, trans-, and post-synaptic) compartments, although they function as a unity, embracing a continuum of micro- and macromolecular interactions. The generation of a nerve impulse represents only a moment in the life of a synapse, but a crucial moment in the succession of events that culminates with the transferral of information.

The pre-synaptic compartment is pictured with two terminals that liberate different substances («circles» and «hexagons»). Following the terminology proposed by BAR-CHAS et al. (1978), we shall call these substances «neuroregulators,» defined as compounds «... that play a key role in communication among nerve cells» (p.964). These can be divided into «neurotransmitters,» «... those which convey information between adjacent nerve cells» (p.964) and «neuromodulators,» «... those which amplify or dampen neuronal activity» (p.964).

The glia and extracellular space are represented within the trans-synaptic compartment, although the latter extends to all areas. The post-synaptic compartment is composed of a neuron with membrane receptors and an apparatus for protein synthesis linked to nuclear post-transcriptional processes.

Several examples of drugs that act at one or more of the defined levels of the synapse will be given. A more detailed explanation of this model is presently in preparation.

I. Pre-synaptic compartment

1. *Axonal transport.* The longitudinal translocation of substances along nerve fibers is a bi-directional phenomenon of varying velocity (see LUBIŃSKA, 1975). It is possible that by means of this process, complex molecules synthesized in the cell body may be transported to the periphery (e.g., nerve growth factor, NGF, and other trophic factors). Colchicine and diphtheria toxin are among the agents that block axonal transport (see LUBIŃSKA, 1975).

2. *Synthesis of neuroregulator(s)*. Organelles such as the mitochondria, endoplasmic reticulum, ribosomes, etc. participate in neuroregulator synthesis. Production can be increased by the administration of precursors of the neuroregulator (e.g., L-DOPA, 5-hydroxytryptophan, choline), or inhibited with enzymatic blockers such as α-methyl-p-tyrosine for catecholamines, styryl pyridine derivatives for acetylcholine, p-chlorophenylalanine for serotonin, etc. (see COOPER et al., 1978).

Based on recent evidence indicating the presence of two or more neuroregulators in the same synaptic terminal (HÖK-FELT et al., 1978), the coexistence of different enzymatic apparatus and, therefore, of possible interactions between them can be proposed at this level.

3. *Storage of neuroregulator(s)*. GRAY (1973) has demonstrated the existence of several types of synaptic vesicles. The storage of neuroregulators in the pre-synaptic compartment, besides constituting the largest pool of these substances, is also a step in the «maturation» of the transmitter (DAHL-STROM, 1973). The size of the pool does not only depend upon *de novo* synthesis, but on the reuptake of neurotransmitters from the synaptic cleft as well. Reserpine and tetrabenazine interfere with the incorporation of neurotransmitters in the synaptic vesicles (CARLSSON, 1965).

4. *Release of neuroregulator(s)*. Release of neuroregulators can take place by the emptying of the contents of the synaptic vesicles or by the release of free molecules found in the cytoplasm. It can occur in the absence of a nerve impulse (KATZ, 1969), but more commonly is a consequence of the arrival of an impulse. Several agents that can inhibit release are the toxin produced by *C. botulinum* in the case of acetylcholine, and lithium for norepinephrine (see COOPER et al., 1978). Amphetamine is reported to increase the release of catecholamines from the presynaptic terminal (CARLSSON, 1965).

5. *Presynaptic receptor and reuptake of neuroregulator(s)*. The receptors located at the level of the presynaptic membrane can be «autoreceptors,» controlling the release of a neurotransmitter (LANGER, 1977), or responsive to sub-

stances released by other cells. We have also included in this model hypothetical receptors to molecules released from the post-synaptic compartment (Fig.1, 12, 13). There is recent evidence that LSD interferes with the autoreceptors of serotonergic cells (AGHAJANIAN & HAIGLER, 1975). Among the inhibitors of the catecholamine reuptake process are cocaine, amphetamine, and tricyclic antidepressant compounds (COOPER et al., 1978).

6. *Presynaptic interaction mediated by neurotransmitter(s)*. Neurotransmitter-mediated presynaptic interactions can be of an excitatory or inhibitory nature (see ECCLES, 1964). In the model, a neurotransmitter from nerve ending A is represented as occupying receptors in the terminal of B, and vice versa. If presynaptic inhibition involves a reduction in neurotransmitter release, then these receptors are closely related to the processes of synthesis and storage in the ending where they are located.

7. *Presynaptic terminal-glia interaction mediated by neurotransmitter(s)*. Presynaptic terminal-glia interactions have recently been demonstrated with the electron microscope (TUSQUES et al., 1976) in human cerebral cortex and are reported to have the form of «typical synapses.» Even though no pharmacological effect has been demonstrated at this level, it represents an obvious possibility for further investigation.

8. *Presynaptic terminal-glia interaction mediated by peptide(s)*. There is evidence that protein material is transferred between neurons and glial cells (LASEK et al., 1977) and that the glia respond to the administration of NGF (TURNER & GLAZE, 1978). Glia also participate in the inactivation of neurotransmitters released into the synaptic cleft.

II. Trans-synaptic compartment

9. *Extracellular space.* Although some authors consider the extracellular space to be almost non-existent at the level of the CNS, it is nevertheless visible under the electron microscope and is sufficiently large to fill nutritional, hydroelectrolytic,

and hormonal requirements. Inactivation of neurotransmitters can also take place in this region; for example, COMT (catechol-0-methyltransferase), an inactivating enzyme for catecholamines, is probably located here.

10. *Glia-neuron and glia-extracellular space interactions.* There exists a close metabolic relationship between the glia and neurons (WATSON, 1976); for example, it has been demonstrated that the development of the neuroglia keeps pace with that of the dendritic tree. This might suggest that the glia have a stabilizing role in newly formed synapses.

The best known functions of the neuroglia are those related to nutrition, protection, immunization, isolation (by means of the myelin), and control of blood flow. These functions are mainly carried out in an indirect manner. We propose, however, that direct inter-relationships can take place through the mediation of simple (e.g., neurotransmitters) or complex (e.g., peptides) molecules, whose effects can be detected at the neuronal level (e.g., see GROSSMAN & SEREGIN, 1977) or extraneuronally, either in normal or lesioned systems (see Chapter 6 by BRAILOWSKY in this volume).

III. Post-synaptic compartment

11. *Occupation of the receptor.* For simplicity, the postsynaptic membrane has been drawn here with only two types of receptors, corresponding to the neuroregulators contained in endings A and B. However, this is not meant to imply that there could not be many more; in fact, we can imagine this membrane as a harlequin's suit, composed of many pieces of cloth of various colors, each one of which represents a different receptor.

The events at the synapse which proceed from the occupation of these receptors have classically been described at the ionic level: depolarization or hyperpolarization of the postsynaptic membrane. Nevertheless, there exists another class of effects with longer time constants (see Fig. 1, 11a–f). These processes are hypothetical, although there exists experimental evidence supporting the presence of some of them (e.g.,

GREENGARD, 1976; AGRANOFF et al., 1978). Note that all the reactions have been represented as reversible and bi-directional.

Among the processes engendered by the occupation of the receptor are those linked to phosphorylation (NATHANSON, 1977) and protein synthesis. They are mediated by «transduction factors» (TFs), proposed molecules that would translate the signals generated by the presence of an agonist or antagonist at the membrane receptor into the language of the cell. A TF corresponds to the so-called second messenger described by KLAINER et al. (1962).

M1, M2, and M3 would be cytoplasmic messenger molecules, or even trophic factors, involved with neuromodulation. Each messenger is related to a different neuronal function: M1 with the occupation of the postsynaptic receptor; M2 with the control of the density and specificity of the postsynaptic receptor; and M3 with the release of neuromodulators from the presynaptic (e.g., trophic factors, see 1 in text) or postsynaptic (see 5 in text) membranes. This model includes a representation of the control which the cell nucleus may exert over the structural quality and density of the membrane receptors (e), as well as the hypothetical possibility that there exists a *postsynaptic* release of molecules that regulate the activity of the glia and/or presynaptic nerve endings (Fig. 1, 12, 13). Included in Table I are some characteristic examples of agonists and antagonists of different postsynaptic brain receptors. This list, however, is far from being exhaustive.

Table I. Agonists and antagonists of various postsynaptic brain receptors[1].

Neuroregulator	Agonist	Antagonist
Acetylcholine: nicotinic receptor	Nicotine	Curare
muscarinic receptor	Muscarine	Scopolamine
Dopamine	Apomorphine	Haloperidol
Serotonin	LSD[2]	LSD[2]
GABA	Muscimol	Bicuculline
Enkephalin	Morphine	Naloxone

[1] Data gathered from COOPER et al. (1978).
[2] LSD action depends on dose.

We have sought to illustrate several of the possibilities which exist for the manipulation of synaptic processes by means of drugs, and some of the factors that should be taken into account when explaining the action of drugs in normal or lesioned neuronal systems.

Although complex, this model is only a schematization of part of the reality. In a future article, we shall further explore the synapse in an attempt to frame hypotheses concerning several phenomena such as hypersensitivity, synaptogenesis, tolerance, and dependence.

References

AGHAJANIAN, G.K., HAIGLER, H.J.: Hallucinogenic indoleamines: preferential action upon presynaptic serotonin receptors. Psychopharmacol. Comm. *1*, 619–629, 1975.

AGRANOFF, B.W., BURRELL, H.R., DOKAS, L.A., SPRINGER, A.D.: Progress in biochemical approaches to learning and memory. In: Lipton, M.A., DiMascio, A., Killam, K.F. (Eds.): Psychopharmacology: A Generation of Progress. Raven Press, New York 1978; pp.623–635.

BARCHAS, J.D., AKIL, H., ELLIOT, G.R., HOLMAN, R.B., WATSON, S.J.: Behavioral neurochemistry: neuroregulators and behavioral states. Science *200*, 964–973, 1978.

CARLSSON, A.: Drugs which block the storage of 5-hydroxy-tryptamine and related amines. In: Eichler, O., Farah, A. (Eds.): Handbook of Experimental Pharmacology. Springer, Berlin 1965; pp.529–592.

COOPER, J.R., BLOOM, F.E., ROTH, R.H.: The Biochemical Basis of Neuropharmacology, 3rd ed. Oxford University Press, New York 1978; p.272.

DAHLSTRÖM, A.: Aminergic transmission. Introduction and short review. Brain Res. *62*, 441–460, 1973.

ECCLES, J.C.: The Physiology of Synapses. Springer, Berlin 1964; p.316.

GRAY, E.G.: The cytonet, plain and coated vesicles, reticulosomes, multivesicular bodies and nuclear pores. Brain Res. *62*, 329–335, 1973.

GREENGARD, P.: Possible role for cyclic nucleotides and phosphorylated membrane proteins in postsynaptic actions of neurotransmitters. Nature *260*, 101–108, 1976.

GROSSMAN, R.G., SEREGIN, A.: Glial-neuron interaction demonstrated by the injection of Na^+ and Li^+ into cortical glia. Science *195*, 196–198, 1977.

HÖKFELT, T., LJUNGDAHL, Å., ELDE, R.P., NILSSON, G., TERENIUS, L., GOLDSTEIN, M., STEINBUSCH, H., VERHOFSTAD, A.: Interdependence of neurotransmitters and systems – morphological basis. Abst. 1313, Proc. 7th Inter.Congr.Pharmacol., Paris, July 16–21, 1978; p.508.

KATZ, B.: The Release of Neural Transmitter Substances. Liverpool University Press, Liverpool 1969; p.60.

KLAINER, L.M., CHI, Y.-M., FRIEDBERG, S.L., RALL, T.W., SUTHERLAND, E.: Adenyl cyclase. IV. The effects of neurohormones on the formation of adenosine 3′, 5′-phosphate by preparations from brain and other tissues. J.Biol.Chem. *237,* 1239–1243, 1962.

LANGER, S.Z.: Presynaptic receptors and their role in the regulation of transmitter release. Brit.J.Pharmacol. *60,* 481–497, 1977.

LASEK, R.J., GAINER, H., BARKER, J.L.: Cell-to-cell transfer of glial proteins to the squid giant axon. J.Cell Biol. *74,* 501–523, 1977.

LUBIŃSKA, L.: On axoplasmic flow. In: Pfeiffer, C.C., Smythies, J.R. (Eds.): International Review of Neurobiology, vol.17. Academic Press, New York 1975; pp.241–296.

NATHANSON, J.A.: Cyclic nucleotides and nervous system functions. Physiol.Rev. *57,* 157–256, 1977.

TURNER, J.E., GLAZE, K.A.: Glial reaction to nerve growth factor in the regenerating optic nerve of the newt *(Triturus viridiscens).* Exp.Neurol. *59,* 190–201, 1978.

TUSQUES, J., GEORGE, Y., ROCH, M.: Mise en évidence du synapses typiques entre neurones et oligodendrocytes dans l'écorce cérébrale humaine. C.R. Acad.Sci. (Paris) *283,* 1747–1749, 1976.

WATSON, W.E.: Cell Biology of the Brain. Chapman and Hall, Cambridge, U.K. 1976; p.527.

Brain plasticity as a basis for therapeutic procedures

P. BACH-Y-RITA

In an evaluation of the theoretical bases for the development of therapeutic procedures for brain-injured patients, plasticity is a prominent factor. In each of the previous chapters this is evident. Although this factor has long been recognized (e.g., BETHE, 1930), it has been increasingly appreciated in the last few years (e.g., BACH-Y-RITA, 1972; STEIN et al., 1974; FINGER, 1978; CLEMENTE, 1976; COTMAN, 1978). Therapeutic procedures that improve function must produce changes at some level of the central nervous system (e.g., ROSENZWEIG, Chapter 5). A particularly important demonstration has been provided by the experiments of CHOW and STEWART (1972) on visually deprived cats. They repeated the studies of previous authors who had reported that permanent behavioral and neural deficits follow deprivation during certain developmental stages. However, CHOW and STEWART (1972) added extremely vigorous training to the research protocol. Their procedures included positive and negative rewards. They found that the forced usage aided in the return of function. They not only obtained an important measure of behavioral recovery, but were able to demonstrate concomitant neural changes in the lateral geniculate nucleus and in the visual cortex. Speculation that comparable neural changes will be found accompanying restitution of function in stroke and head injury victims who have undergone comprehensive rehabilitation programs is in order.

In this chapter, I shall briefly review the concept of plasticity, followed by a description of some of our studies and other human studies in this area, and I shall attempt to relate plasticity to the development of therapeutic procedures. The last section will examine some little-understood factors, such as motivation and the mind-body interactions, since these must be considered in the evaluation of therapeutic procedures that produce functional changes and reveal brain plasticity. Much of what is summarized here has been published elsewhere (BACH-Y-RITA, 1967, 1971, 1972, 1975a, 1975b, 1976a, 1976b, in press; BACH-Y-RITA et al., 1969).

Brain plasticity refers to the adaptive capacities of the central nervous system – its ability to modify its own structural organization and functioning. It is an adaptive response to functional demand. It requires feedback on whether or not environmental demands are being met. Plasticity permits enduring functional changes to take place. It is one of the two fundamental properties of the nervous system; the other is its excitability, which relates to rapid changes leaving no trace in the nervous system (KONORSKI, 1961).

BETHE (1930) considered plasticity a general principle of living organisms: the ability to adapt to changes and to meet the dangers of life. It is the capacity of the central nervous system to reorganize following insult and to restore adequate function.

The question of CNS plasticity is intimately linked with concepts of cerebral localization, the neural substrate of the various functions of the CNS. Some functions are more localized than others. For example, LURIA (1963) considers that the localization of such processes as visual and auditory perception in circumscribed sensory areas is less likely than the localization of the respiratory or patellar reflex. However, he notes that in the cortical representation of the special senses such as vision and audition, the cortical projections are only a small part of the functional system of that part of the brain. The high specificity of the neuronal structures that project a particular receptor system to the cortex underlies the fact that lesions in these areas often lead to irreversible defects, and compensation is possible only within very narrow limits. This discussion on plasticity will be concerned principally with the restoration of function following a CNS lesion.

Early studies on CNS plasticity

In 1842 FLOURENS (cited in CLARKE & O'MALLEY, 1968) noted that destruction of isolated areas of the cerebral hemispheres in birds produced behavioral defects, but a short time after the injury, normal behavior returned. GOLTZ (cited in CLARKE & O'MALLEY, 1968) in the last quarter of the 19th century extirpated several cortical areas in dogs, producing defects, but noted that with the passage of time marked restoration of function occurred. In work spanning the end of the last century and the beginning of this century, BETHE (1930), a student of GOLTZ, developed concepts of CNS plasticity that have influenced many other workers. One of his demonstrations involved the assessment of functional reorganization following removal of one, two, or three limbs of an amphibian. The animal continued to move about by recoordinating in a new manner. BETHE's work on plasticity has led to the conclusion that the high degree of plasticity in man and higher vertebrates is due to dynamic reorganization and adaptation to new circumstances and not to regeneration. Studies demonstrating the «unmasking» of previously unrecognized pathways following peripheral nerve or central nervous system lesions (WALL, Chapter 3), and the demonstration of synaptically weak polysensory pathways in the visual cortex (described below), support this view.

Early in this century, LEYTON & SHERRINGTON (1917) showed that extirpation of cortical motor areas in monkeys produced marked paresis, but over a period of time, recovery occurred. They further showed that ablation of the arm area produced marked motor deficits from which the primate recovered completely in one month, but that reoperation, extending the lesion, did not increase the motor deficit. Two-stage operations removing the arm area of each cortex revealed that recovery from the first lesion was not due to take-over by the corresponding area of the opposite cortex. About the same time, OGDEN & FRANZ (1917) completed an important study on the role of training in functional recovery following destruction of the precentral gyrus in rhesus monkeys.

Similarly, FOERSTER (cited in ZÜLCH, 1969) had long (since

the turn of the century) emphasized the role of physical therapy in effecting recovery from CNS lesions. He further showed that deficits due to lesions in the less highly differentiated parts of the brain, or in which there is a bilateral representation of receptors, show a greater capacity for improvement. FOERSTER was one of the outstanding clinical exponents of CNS plasticity; he, as well as BETHE (1930) and others, considered that recovery of function takes place by means of the reorganization of the remaining parts of the CNS.

In the second quarter of this century, several clinical studies on muscle relocation demonstrated the CNS capacity to reorganize complex reflexes and motor functions. For example, WEISS & BROWN (1941) transposed the biceps femoris muscle (a flexor) to the extensor side of a knee joint to substitute for the weakened or lost action of a paralyzed quadricepts muscle. Initially, the muscle contracted only in the flexor phase, but «... surprisingly few trials were required to make the transplant suddenly contract in the extensor phase, too». After further trials, the muscle operated only the extensor phase. Even then, however, temporary relapses into the old flexor association occur repeatedly, even years after the operation. These relapses seem to be favored by fatigue, lack of concentration, automaticity of movement, etc. WEISS & BROWN (1941) suggested that the adjusted use of the transplant is not based on the substitution of a permanent extensor association for its former flexor association in the elementary motor mechanisms, but rather on the development in higher centers of a new type of action which can effectively override the innate coordinative associations without abolishing them.

For many years studies with stroke and brain-injured patients have revealed unexpected and unexplained recovery that, in retrospect, could be interpreted in terms of brain plasticity. However, plasticity was, in general, not considered. On the contrary, the brain was considered to be a rigid, unchanging organ. CLEMENTE (1976) has pointed out that although everyone admitted that an individual could learn, and thus show functional plasticity, learning was considered an abstract function, related to the mind and not the brain. Once the physical neural patterns of the nervous system had developed, i.e., once the fiber connections had become established, alterations in neuronal geometry were not considered possible. CLEMENTE considers that a change in thinking occurred as the gap between the mind and the body began to close. «The so-called structure of the mind had never been considered rigid, only the structure of the brain. It followed naturally that since the brain was the organ of the mind, and that since the brain was composed of cells, that plasticity could only be the result of cellular events in the central nervous system.« CLEMENTE suggests that the ambient aura for acceptance of the concept of central nervous system plasticity really developed as a post-World War II phenomenon. He considers that this, together with the recent re-evaluation of old anatomical evidence and new experimental evidence (especially anatomical, physiological, and biochemical) for plasticity, has altered our views.

One particularly important change in the concept of the brain as a malleable organ resulted from the demonstration that, although the individual brain cells did not regenerate, the cell *processes,* axons and dendrites, were highly responsive to functional demand (some of this work has been reviewed in Chapters 3 and 5). CRAGG (1968) has pointed out that, in the rat visual cortex, cell bodies occupy only 3% of the volume of the cortex. Thus 97% of the cortex is made up primarily by dendrites, axons and glia. The large difference between the weight of the brain at birth and at maturity is due to the development of these three structures, since the number of cells does not increase. Figure 1 is a schematic representation of the changes in axon development and dendritic arborization during maturation of human cortex, and the reversal of this growth with senescence (SHEIBEL, 1977). Note particularly that at maximum development, the dendritic tree is full, with horizontal components and with many dendritic spines (small spurs that look like thorns arising from the dendrites). The horizontal components allow for interaction with other cortical cells, and the dendritic spines are full of synaptic connections to other cells. There is evidence that the development of dendrites and dendritic spines, as well as axons and synapses,

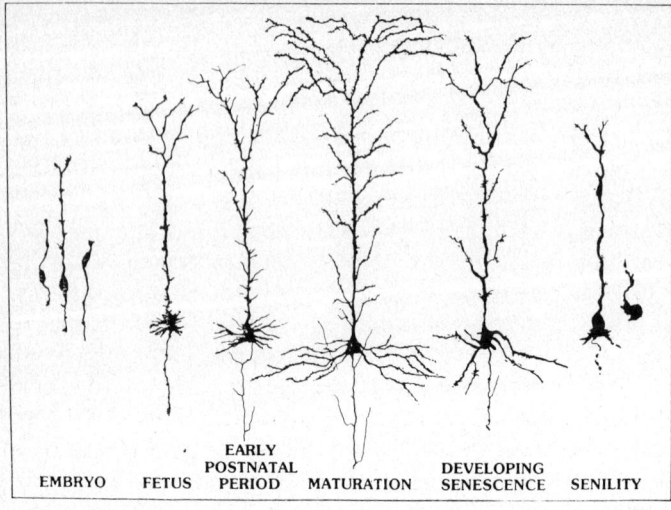

Figure 1. A schematic representation of the changes in axon development and dendritic arborization during maturation of human cortex and the reversal of this growth with senescence (SCHEIBEL, 1977).

depends on functional demand (reviewed in BACH-Y-RITA, 1972). In a recent study of plasticity in the mature and aged human brain, dendritic trees were shown to be more extensive in aged (av. age 79.6) than in adult (av. age 52.1) brains. This suggests a system in which one population of neurons dies and regresses while another survives and grows. This late growth is not found in demented persons (BUELL & COLEMAN, 1979).

Human brain plasticity studies

In previous chapters, considerable evidence for brain plasticity has been presented. In this chapter, further evidence from our laboratories will be discussed, followed by other particularly pertinent human studies.

1. Sensory substitution studies

A person who has suffered the total loss of a sensory modality has, indirectly, suffered a brain lesion. In the absence of the modality, behavior and neural function must be reorganized. We have carried out extensive studies with blind and deaf subjects to test the extent of the brain's ability to reorganize functionally. Our principal work has been with congenitally blind persons: these were considered to be «natural» experiments in whom the major source of afferent information had been eliminated before they had the opportunity to develop the mechanisms for the analysis of visual information.

We developed a tactile vision substitution system (TVSS) to deliver visual information to the brain via arrays of stimulators in contact with one of several parts of the body (abdomen, back, thigh). Optical images are picked up by a TV camera and transduced into a form of energy (vibratory or direct electrical stimulation) that can be mediated by the skin receptors. The visual information reaches the perceptual levels for analysis and interpretation via somatosensory pathways and structures. After sufficient training with the TVSS, including the motor control needed to direct the camera towards the desired visual field, our subjects report experiencing the image in space, instead of on the skin. They quickly learn to make perceptual judgments using visual means of analysis, such as perspective, parallax, looming and zooming, and depth judgments.

Figure 2 shows a blind subject using a TVSS. Our studies with the TVSS have been extensively described (BACH-Y-RITA, 1972; in press; BACH-Y-RITA et al., 1969; COLLINS & BACH-Y-RITA, 1973; WHITE et al., 1970) and will not be repeated here.

The tactile vision substitution system studies have demonstrated that the brain is sufficiently plastic to reorganize function to utilize the information from sensory substitution systems. However, the neural mechanisms underlying the plastic changes in sensory substitution are not known at present. One study from our laboratory has demonstrated that blind persons with extensive tactile training show consistent differences from sighted persons in the somatosensory evoked po-

231

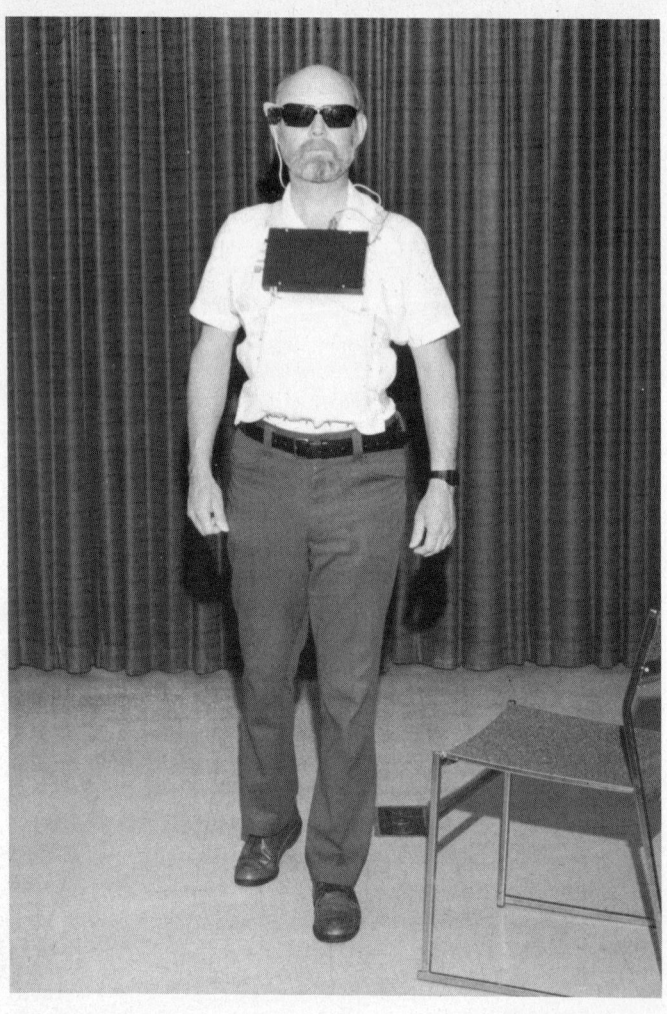

Figure 2. A portable tactile vision substitution system (TVSS). the television camera is mounted on the frame of a pair of glasses (upper left). The black box across his chest contains the commutator, to electronically convert the TV signals to tactile stimuli, delivered to the skin of the abdomen through a 1032-point array of stimulators (courtesy of Dr. C.C.COLLINS).

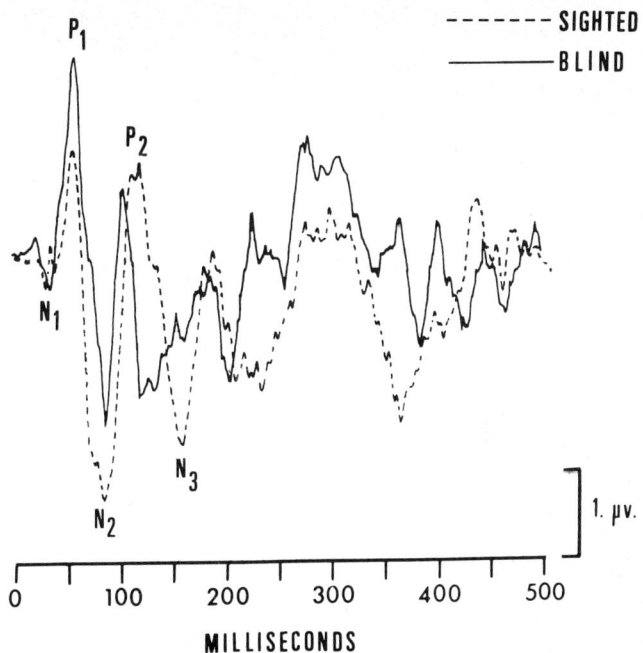

Figure 3. The somatosensory evoked responses of a blind subject (solid line) and a sighted subject (dashed line). The stimulus was delivered to a finger tip in both subjects.

tential (FEINSOD et al., 1973). The stimulus was delivered to the finger, and the evoked potential was recorded over the somatosensory cortex. Figure 3 shows the overlapped evoked potentials of a blind subject (dashed line) and a sighted subject. The fast initial components (N_1 and P_1) of the sensory evoked response (SER) are regarded as thalamic radiation responses (CRACCO, 1972). Their latencies are thus related to the conduction along peripheral (median) nerve and spinothalamic tracts (PAGNI, 1967), which are not altered by blindness. However, a difference between the blind and sighted subjects is evident at components N_2, P_2, and N_3. In each case, the component occurs earlier in the blind subject. Figure 4 shows the results for all subjects. The latency of N_2 was

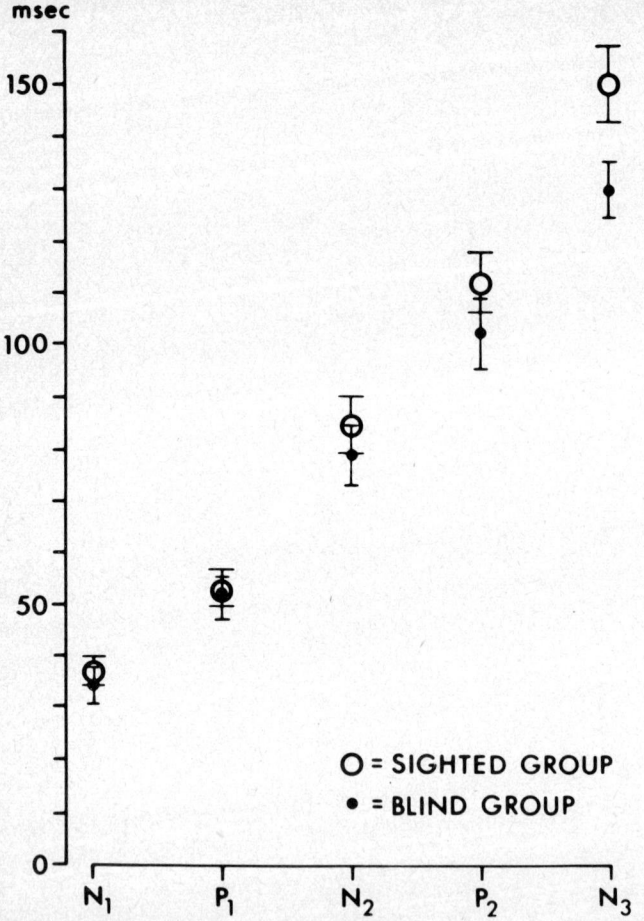

Figure 4. The somatosensory evoked response latencies for all the blind (solid circles) and sighted (open circles) subjects studied. In each case the stimulus was delivered to a finger tip (FEINSOD et al., 1973).

shorter by 6%, of P_2 by 9% and of N_3 by 13% in the blind subjects.

The significant shortening of the late N_3 component may be comparable to the late waves of similar latencies which were found by several authors to be sensitive to attention, barbiturates, and sleep. The late components have been considered to be maximally affected by any procedure that alters the perceptual organization of the subject (discussed in FEINSOD et al., 1973). All the previous studies referred to changes in the amplitudes of the wave components. We suggested that the marked differences in the latencies of the N_3 component might reflect faster processing of the tactile stimulus in the trained blind subjects (FEINSOD et al., 1973).

We have developed sensory substitution systems for other disabilities. The tactile auditory substitution system presents words and phrases connected to touch patterns via a 32-stimulator electrical stimulation unit. The sound information appears as flowing dynamic patterns on the skin. The system is presently being tested with profoundly deaf children (SAUNDERS et al., 1978).

Electromyographic (EMG) sensory feedback (also called «EMG biofeedback») is another example of sensory substitution. In this case, the visual or auditory display of the EMG data is substituting for the absent or altered proprioception. BRUDNY et al. (1976) have reviewed the studies using this technique (which they call «sensory feedback therapy») in patients with various manifestations of disturbed neuromotor control. They have analyzed its application in 114 of their cases, including 45 hemiparetics. They obtained favorable results, such as the breaking up of pathological synergy patterns with the return of patterned function. The patients with a greater degree of sensory loss usually responded in a more rapid manner. They concluded that the audio-visual sensory feedback from integrated EMG can be considered as a temporary substitute for the proprioceptive internal feedback loops; this external loop augments or restores the sensorimotor interaction of the closed loop system of voluntary patterned movements. They consider that the sensory feedback therapy allowed the transfer of motor control from indirect exteroceptive feedback to direct feedback, thus allowing lasting functional improvement in their patients. BRUDNY and his collaborators have recently concluded that the results obtained with hemiparetic patients treated with EMG sensory

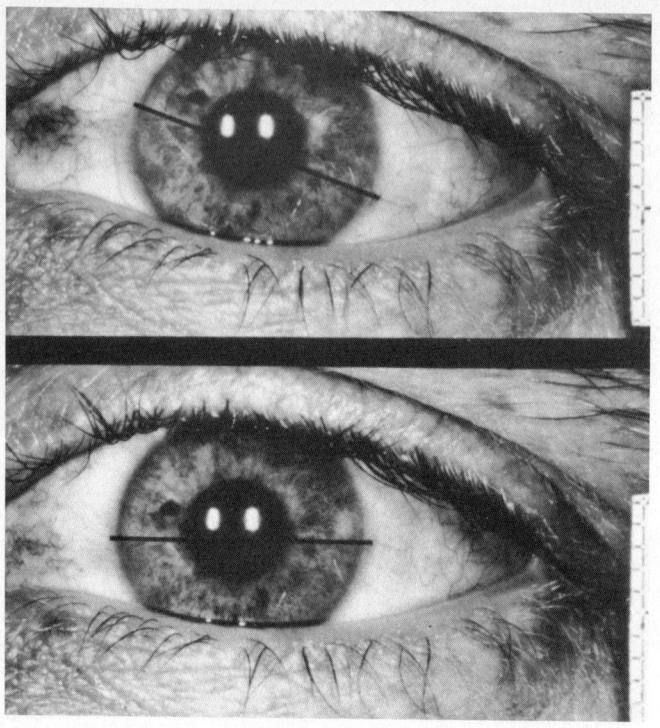

Figure 5. Photographs showing a tonic voluntary cyclotorsion of 20°. Bars drawn across the irises demonstrate the torsion that is measured from photographic displacement of two identifiable limbal-scleral blood vessel junctions (BALLIET & NAKAYAMA, 1978).

feedback justify «... a more optimistic perspective regarding the outlook for recovery of function in the hemiparetic upper extremity» (BRUDNY et al., 1979).

In our laboratories, BALLIET & NAKAYAMA (1978) have explored the ability to develop new motor control by training normal subjects to produce a voluntary movement that is not present in the absence of specific training. By means of a visual feedback technique, human subjects were trained to make large conjugate cyclorotary eye movements (rotation of each eye around an anterior-posterior axis) at will (Figure 5). The range of movement increased with training at a rate of approximately 0.8° per hour of practice, reaching 30° at the end of training. The subjects learned to make saccadic and pursuit cyclorotary movements. Control experiments indicate that all of the movements were voluntary, with no significant visual induction. With extended practice, large torsional movements could be made without any visual feedback. The authors concluded that the emergence of voluntary torsion through training demonstrates that the oculomotor system has more plasticity than has generally been assumed, reopening the issue as to whether other movements could also be trained to alleviate the symptoms of strabismus.

2. Vestibular and limb control studies

MELVILL JONES & GONSHOR (1975) have demonstrated that it is possible to change the human vestibulo-ocular response (VOR) by inducing vision reversal during head rotation. This is considerd a primitive reflex, relating to the interaction between the vestibular and ocular interaction; the main vestibular source of reflex drive to the muscles moving the eye originates in the rotation-sensing semicircular canals of the vestibular mechanical end organs. MELVILL JONES & GONSHOR investigated VOR changes due to prolonged vision-reversal, by using goggles, fitted with dove prisms causing reversal in the horizontal, but not vertical, plane. They were continuously worn during normal movements throughout all waking hours for periods up to 28 days. After about two weeks of continuous vision reversal, the vestibulo-ocular response recorded in the dark was not merely attenuated, but had become effectively completely reversed. MELVILL JONES & GONSHOR (1975) stated «... one may guess that the goal towards which plastic change was driven amounted to re-acquisition of automatic image stabilization by means of the vestibulo-ocular reflex.» They concluded that in addition to «hard wired» neuronal connections, other central elements permit substantial levels of goal-directed plastic change when such change is functionally called for.

Limb movement in zero gravity (as encountered by astronauts in outer space) is altered due to the decreased load of a weightless arm. GUITTON (1975) has pointed out that the brain must reformulate the templates which are to anticipate the new sensory and motor events. This does occur, and astronauts do adapt. It takes one to two weeks in space for this adaption; no amount of prior training or earth can help. GUITTON (1975) considers that the templates are specific and must be elaborated in situ.

3. Recovery from stroke

Stroke patients occasionally recover far more function than could have been predicted. But in such cases, there is rarely knowledge of the exact pathological lesion, and recovery is often ascribed to various benign factors, such as reabsorption of edema (although restitution of function occurring later than the first two months cannot be explained in this way (BRODAL, 1972)), or else the original insult is considered to have been relatively minor. Similarly, it has been difficult to evaluate the efficacy of stroke rehabilitation programs in producing actual recovery or reorganization of function.

The case described below offered an unusual opportunity to relate brain plasticity to recovery of function following a stroke, due to the conjunction of various factors: a cerebral vascular insult in a previously intact elderly person; an intensive therapy program; a high degree of motivation and family involvement; an excellent recovery over a period of several years; a post-mortem examination following death, seven years after the cerebral vascular accident, from an unrelated cause.

The patient was a 65 year old college professor (my father) who recovered following a brainstem infarct and returned to full-time work 3 years after the event (at age 68). He led an ac-

---

Figure 6. A section from the brain of a 72 year old man who had recovered from a stroke (pontine infarct) 7 years previously.

a) A $1 \times 1 \times 0.5$ cm irregular focus of old cystic encephalomalacia is seen in the left half of the rostral basis pontis which extended from near the midline to within 0.5 cm of the lateral margin of this structure.

b) Microscopically, the lesion in the left basis pontis is seen to be totally cystic in its central portion, with no viable tissue remaining (AGUILAR, 1969).

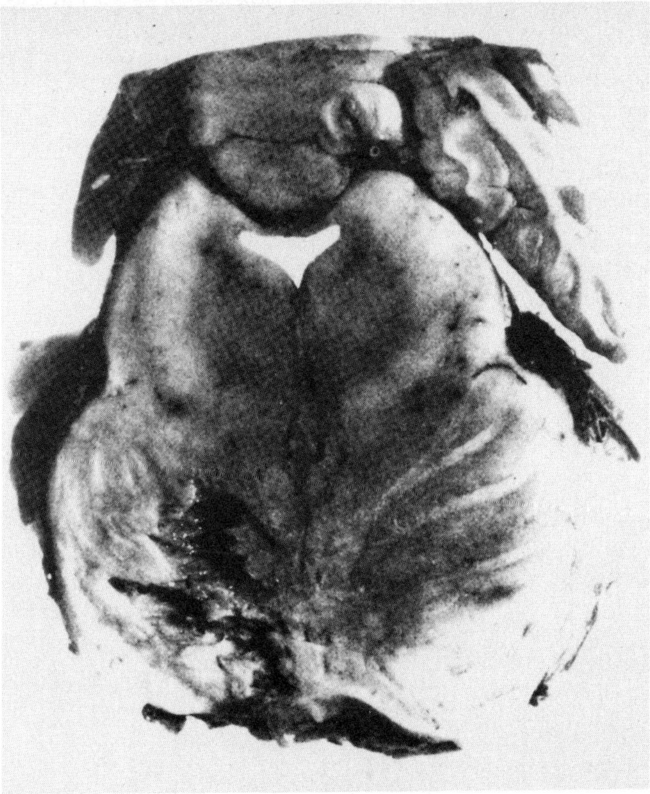

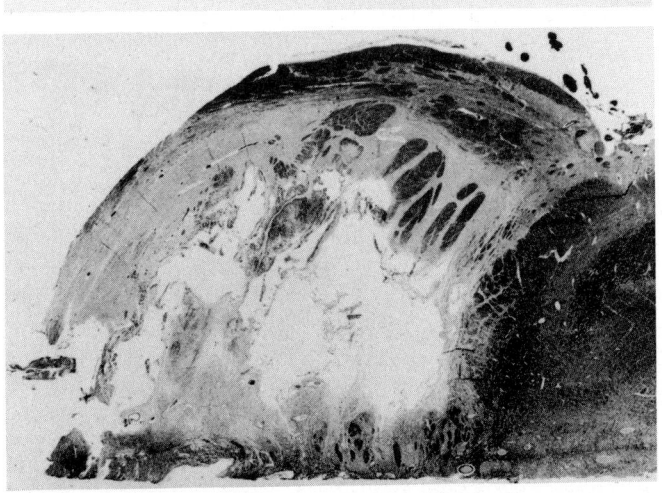

tive life until his death at age 72 of a myocardial infarction, which occurred during a mountain hiking trip at 9000 feet altitude. Autopsy revealed the existence of major neural damage which had occurred at the time of the stroke 7 years previously. There was a $1 \times 1 \times 0.5$ cm irregular focus of old cystic encephalomalacia in the left half of the rostral basis pontis which extended from near the midline to within 0.5 cm of the lateral margin of this structure (Figure 6a). Distal to this lesion the pyramidal tract in the left medulla oblongata was severely atrophic, appearing shrunken and gray on coronal section. Microscopically, the lesion in the left basis pontis was seen to be totally cystic in its central portion, with no viable neural tissue remaining (Figure 6b). A few intact longitudinally coursing fiber bundles remained in the medialmost and lateralmost margins of the area, but the major portion of the left basis pontis showed nearly total demyelination and axonal degeneration of its fiber tracts, with large numbers of periodic acid-Schiff-positive gitter cells scattered through the lesion.

Distally, the ipsilateral pyramidal tract in the medulla oblongata showed severe demyelination and gliosis (Figure 7a), with only sparsely scattered intact fibers remaining. Below the decussation of the pyramids, the right lateral and left ventral corticospinal tracts in the cervical spinal cord showed similar degenerative changes (Figure 7b) with, however, approximately 3% of the myelinated axons remaining, widely scattered. The demyelinating and atrophic changes were limited to the corticospinal pathways of the lower brainstem and spinal cord. There were no changes in the corticospinal pathway rostral to the lesion (AGUILAR, 1969).

The recovery in this case proceeded over a period of 5 years, during which time the patient was engaged in an active home therapy program and, during the first part, a three-hour per week physical therapy program. Fine movements, such as button closing and fast typing, were regained. The patient was extremely active in all phases of his own rehabilitation program, and was willing to work hard for many hours a day, for a few years. Many of the specific tasks he thought of himself. For example, several months after his injury, he de-

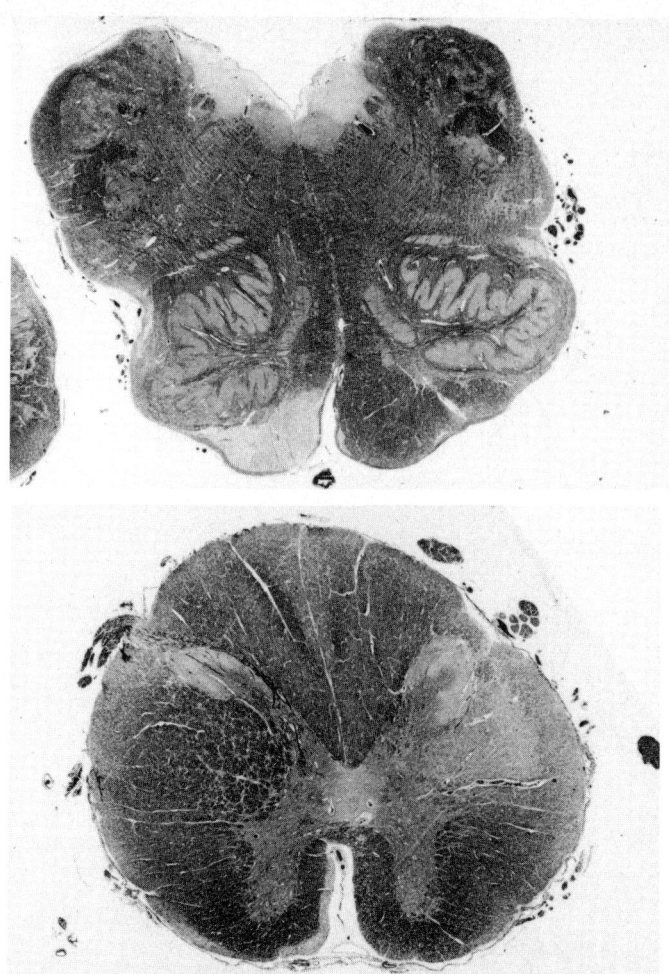

Figure 7. The same patient as in Fig. 6.

a) the ipsilateral pyramidal tract showed severe demyelinization and gliosis.

b) Below the decussation of the pyramids, the right lateral and left ventral corticospinal tracts in the cervical spinal cord showed similar degenerative changes (AGUILAR, 1969).

241

cided he would wash the dinner dishes daily. Initially, this took a couple of hours. He would keep his involved (right) hand in the warm dishwater and progressively, over the next few months, this hand was able to participate more and more actively in the process of washing the dishes. A comparable self-designed task was typewriting. Although he could write with his left hand, he refused to do so. Several months after the accident, he noted that he could lift his arm over the typewriter, visually position his arm so that the middle finger was above the desired key, and then drop his arm, striking the key. Thus, using very gross movements, and with many errors, he was able to begin to type. He practiced at this continuously and progressively was able to include individual wrist and, later, finger movements, and his typewriting speed increased markedly over the succeeding year.

The program was not formally documented and thus the conclusions are of limited value. Furthermore, some brain-stem lesions have a better prognosis for functional recovery than cortical lesions. Nevertheless, several points emerge:

1. Functional recovery can occur even when the lesion is massive and the age is advanced. The functional recovery in the presence of the damage demonstrated at autopsy is evidence of a high level of plasticity, and requires interpretation in the framework of mechanisms discussed previously (BACH-Y-RITA, 1972) and in this volume by WALL (Chapter 3). It is possible that the approximately 3% of remaining normal fibers served as the basis of reorganization. If this were so, it would suggest that the dendritic arborizations of the remaining normal cells must have established more functional connections with other cells above the level of the pontine lesion, and the long axons must have established more functional connections to interneurons and motor cells below the level of the lesion. This could be by the same means that led to the «unmasking» of pathways in WALL's (Chapter 3) studies. The studies of GALAMBOS et al. (1967) on the recovery of visual evoked response amplitude after optic tract lesion (see below) support the suggestion that a great potential exists for «unmasking» pathways.

2. Motivation was a major factor in the recovery. Important also was the ability to concentrate on what he was doing.

3. A program that approximates real life activities and pre-lesion interests was of particular value.

4. Non-professional therapy can be successful. Professional therapy is very expensive and thus is not available to all. When it is available, relatively few hours of individual therapy are feasible. In the case described above, home therapy was directed by one of the patient's sons (then a medical student and now a psychiatrist). In the case of the actress Patricia Neal, non-professional therapy was directed by her husband, and included a group of friends and relatives. It was continued by another volunteer, who later described her methods (GRIFFITH, 1970). The Frenkel methodology of rehabilitation that began almost 100 years ago and has had a great influence on the field of rehabilitation originated from the casual observations of a self-rehabilitated patient (LICHT, 1975).

The process of functional reorganization following a stroke may be loosely compared to learning a new language. The central nervous system (CNS) substrate exists in most humans, but is not called upon unless a need occurs. Motivation and training are necessary: Children learn more quickly and are more able to completely acquire the accent, grammar and subtleties of a language. The absence of learning is *not* prima facie evidence of the absence of the capacity to learn the language: either adequate training or motivation may have been absent, or training may have continued for an insufficient time. Great experience with language training has led to the development of methods that produce highly efficient results. The amount of training required is usually related to age. In fact, young children require no further training than exposure to the language. However, with increasing age, exposure alone is insufficient: Numerous examples exist of immigrants to the USA who, even after 50 years of residence, are unable to speak English.

Although the CNS lesion may not be incompatible with life, the quality of life is certainly reduced unless a considerable amount of functional recovery occurs. Thus, a stroke patient may live at a reduced level for many years with hemiplegia and aphasia. (Comparably, the long-time resident of the USA who has not learned English can exist within his cultural subgroup without being able to participate in many of the activities that surround him.) Each small increment of functional reorganization will improve the quality of his life.

A particular problem in rehabilitation that has not been widely discussed is the last portion of improvement. The major gains in function are usually made early, and small increases in function continue for some time, but often, the efforts cease short of full recovery[1]. My father continued to work hard for relatively small gains even in the fifth post-lesion year, and thus, was able to return to a functional level indistinguishable from normal by the casual observer. Patricia Neal, however, was unwilling to proceed to work for the small gains: «... I got fed up with working so hard. I felt certain that I was as good as I'd ever be. I was about 80% recovered. Still plenty of problems. But I was ready to take a breather. I wanted to give up and lie back and do nothing. And that is exactly what I would have done if Roald (her husband) hadn't made me go on. I had reached the point where so many people stop work and just cruise along (P.NEAL, in GRIFFITH, 1970, p.89).»

The extra effort enabled Patricia Neal, an Academy Awardwinning actress, to recover that last portion of function that permitted her to resume her acting career. However, it is doubtful that a 100% recovery can be obtained after major lesions, such as those suffered by Ms.Neal or the patient described above. BRODAL, who published a neuroanatomical-neurophysiological analysis of his own stroke (BRODAL, 1972) later stated «... there is not a complete recovery even if it may appear so. ... I think, in general, following a stroke, and other brain injuries, there will always be minor sequelae, which an observant patient will notice, but which are not obvious to

---

[1] In experimental psychology, FITTS' law (FITTS, 1964) states that skill increases with practice according to a power function (with a fractional exponent). Thus, after rapid early gains one seems to reach a plateau, but there continues to be improvement with practice – it just occurs more and more slowly.

others and may not be detected in a routine examination.»
(Personal communication, 1976.)

Factors related to reorganization of function

The previous chapters have discussed a number of mechanisms that relate to brain plasticity. However, we are still far from an understanding of the means by which brain function is reorganized after a lesion. Factors that require particular discussion include the following: neural substrate, meaningful therapy, age, time, motivation, environment, and family.

Neural substrate

It is evident from GLEES' studies on hemispherectomy (Chapter 4) that reorganization of function can occur after a great amount of brain has been lost. Animal studies reveal that as little as 2% of remaining neural tissue in a particular system can mediate a high degree of function: GALAMBOS et al. (1967) destroyed up to 98.5% of the optic tract fibers in the cat and a few weeks after the lesions, they found almost normal visual behavior. Pattern discrimination was present and visual-evoked potentials had approximately the same amplitude as pre-operatively. Previously, LASHLEY (1939) had demonstrated that complex visual discrimination and visual behavior could be maintained in the rat if only 2% of the visual cortex remained. In the stroke case mentioned above, microscopic examination of the brainstem revealed that approximately 3% normal-appearing axons remained in the atrophic pyramid, and this may have been a morphological basis of the functional reorganization.

Thus, at least in certain cases, a small amount of remaining nervous tissue may be a sufficient neural substrate. But *how* can this occur? One possibility is suggested by WALL's studies. WALL (Chapter 3) has described his experiments revealing pathways that exist in the normal state, but do not appear to function until «unmasked» by injury. In 1963, we demonstrated the existence of weak non-visual inputs to cells of the cat primary visual cortex. Figure 8 shows histograms of the responses to light, sound, and pinprick. The responses to light were tightly grouped around a mean of 33 milliseconds in latency, while those to sound and pinprick were spread out around means of 63 (sound) and 70 (pinprick) milliseconds (MURATA et al., 1965). Further, the responses to sound and pinprick were less synaptically secure, being less resistant to barbiturate narcosis than the visual responses. These more

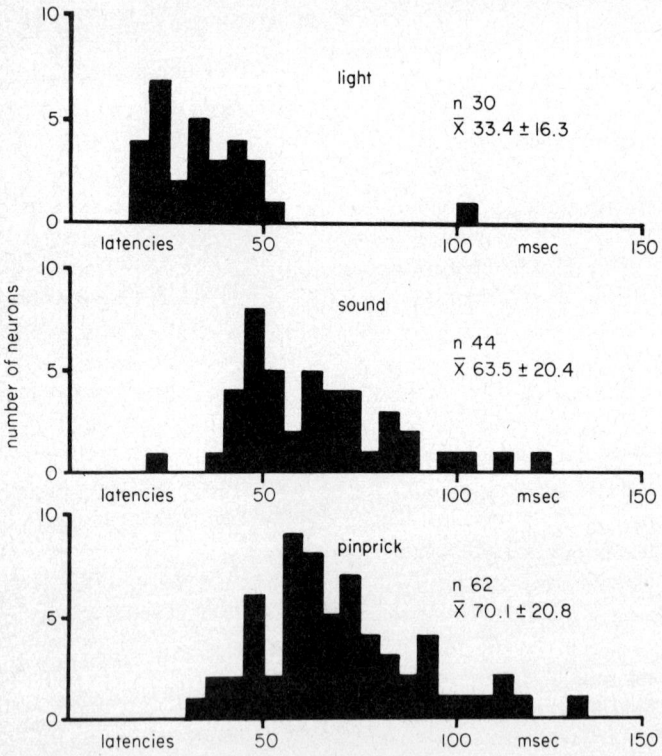

Figure 8. Histograms of latencies in cat visual cortex to visual (light on), acoustic and somesthetic stimuli. Ordinate: number of neurons responding. n = number of neurons treated in these histograms; $\bar{x}$ = mean value of latencies (MURATA et al., 1965).

tenuous pathways may be comparable to the pathways «unmasked» by injury in WALL's studies, and thus may be the type of pathway available for functional reorganization following brain injury.

Professor ALF BRODAL (1972), in an analysis of the mechanisms that may have been involved in the restitution of function following his own stroke, discussed the extremely high specificity of the morphological organization of the nervous system, while at the same time, he recognized the «... fargoing diffuseness in the patterns of innervation.» He notes the «... morphological possibilities for an impulse from a certain part of the brain to be transmitted along circumventional routes of varying complexity to virtually every other part of the central nervous system.» He suggested the possibility that following the lesion, remaining intact and functioning fibers establish new synapses where the destroyed fibers were previously acting. BRODAL (personal communication, 1976) considers that «... motivation is essential, and may in some mystical way influence sprouting.»

A number of studies, some discussed in BACH-Y-RITA (1972), have demonstrated the role of inhibition in learned brain mechanisms. The clinical importance of inhibition had been recognized many years ago. For example, FOERSTER (cited in ZÜLCH, 1969) noted its role in several functions, including the prevention of associated movements. Further, even the concept of «synaptic facilitation» as a basis for learned responses has been seriously challenged by evidence that synaptic use may result in inhibition rather than facilitation. BLISS et al. (1968), in conditioning experiments in isolated cat cortical slabs, have concluded that the great majority of pathways examined must have contained synaptic functions that were less likely to transmit excitation the more often the pathway was used (although some pathways with facilitated synapses were also observed). The majority of cortical synapses displaying plasticity between two cells, X and Y (so arranged that X can excite Y) showed long-lasting changes of conductivity. They were negatively correlated with both the firing rate of X and the use of the XY junction, but were positively correlated with the discharge frequency of Y. However, it should be pointed out that in other cases, synaptic facilitation may play a role in learning.

Similarly, CREUTZFELDT (1975) and his collaborators have studied the function of the intracortical fibers that are formed in great abundance, to determine whether excitatory or inhibitory influences predominated. Intracellular recordings demonstrated that electrical stimulation of cortical afferents produces excitatory, as well as inhibitory, post-synaptic effects on cortical neurons; because of their latency, it was concluded that the inhibitory actions are of intracortical origin, i.e., mediated by cortical interneurons. Such inhibitory effects could also be demonstrated when physiological stimulation was used. CREUTZFELDT (1975) concluded from these and similar studies that «... over a distance of 300–400 microns each cortical neuron is inhibited by its neighbors and that intracortical connections are essentially and dominantly inhibitory.» These and further studies from his laboratory allow him to consider the cortex as an adaptive neuronal network, rather than a fixed-wired system.

A stroke patient experiences an enormous difficulty in initiating movements. With extended practice, often the movements can be performed with less effort. It is possible that mechanisms, such as those described by WALL, are involved in this process. «Unmasking» a pathway means that the pathways become accessible to stimuli. This must be the result of changes in synaptic connectivity which lower the threshold of the relevant synapses. Whether this occurs primarily by changes in neurotransmitter, decreased inhibition, sprouting, or other mechanisms, is not known at this time.

Among those tools that have proved useful for demonstrating the plasticity of neural connections are certain drugs. For example, ADKINS et al. (1966) found, in cats anesthetized with chloralose, that pyramidal stimulation not only increased the size of the cutaneous receptor fields of the recorded neurons, but also revealed responsiveness to sensory modalities that were ineffective in the absence of pyramidal stimulation. ALBE-FESSARD & FESSARD (1963) have summarized a series of experiments showing that administration of chloralose increases the size of cortical evoked potentials in zones of convergence. ROBERTSON (1965) has observed cells in the cat visual cortex before, during, and after administration of thiopental anesthesia and found that the drug increases receptive fields and the types of stimuli to which cells respond; thiopental makes previously unreceptive cells respond to visual stimuli. It is highly unlikely that acutely administered drugs can create new synapses and new pathways. Therefore, it is likely that the drugs are uncovering synapses and pathways that already exist, but are not utilized under normal circumstances (see BACH-Y-RITA, 1972). The pathways may have high thresholds, may be under inhibition in the absence of the drug, or other mechanisms may be responsible for the changes in responsiveness. This drug action is comparable to the «unmasking» described by WALL (Chapter 3).

There is convincing evidence that the brain adjusts to changes in afferent input. For example, DASTUR (1955) studied cutaneous sensitivity in leprosy patients and noted that no sensitivity changes could be observed until a large number of nerve fibers was destroyed. Following damage to sensory pathways, such as in stroke patients, comparable brain mechanisms must aid in recovery of function, enabling the brain to adapt to the altered sensory inflow.

Of course, the studies discussed here reveal reorganization of function when sufficient neural substrate remains after a lesion. The actual percentage necessary may vary from system to system and from function to function. This poses a critical practical problem to rehabilitation clinicians. If the critical minimum neural substrate is not available, no amount of therapy is going to produce functional recovery. Further knowledge in this area would be helpful in selecting candidates for intensive and extensive rehabilitation and would enable the clinician to justify the expenses involved, as well as maintaining the morale of the rehabilitation team.

Meaningful therapy

The primary purpose of this book is to serve as a discussion of theory to aid in developing effective therapeutic procedures.

We do not propose to suggest specific procedures. Other authors (e.g., KOTTKE, 1975) have suggested specific therapy based on neurophysiology. However, a number of specific comments regarding meaningful therapy are in order.

MOORE (Chapter 2) has thoroughly discussed the hierarchical nervous system and has made a cogent case for initiating therapy with the archi, midline system, and specifically, with the neck. She has suggested the possible negative effects of sensory isolation (such as maintaining a patient in a coma in a quiet room with few visitors) versus the possible therapeutic effects of considerable afferent stimulation, for example, having many visitors who speak to the patient even if he does not respond. Another such stimulus is the presence of music (and, she would suggest, music with a «heavy» beat, such as rock music, which may be comparable to the effect of the mother's heartbeat on a fetus). Vestibular and visual stimulation also should be initiated early in the therapy program. It is necessary, however, to consider the possibility that some brain lesions may particularly affect centrifugal sensory cortical mechanisms, the brain's means of selecting important afferent information and filtering out the unimportant information (discussed in BACH-Y-RITA, 1972). In some cases, it may be necessary to restrict afferent information to minimize the confusion caused by the excessive sensory input. LURIA (1963, 1969) recommended that certain brain injured patients be protected against strong stimuli for a period of time. Furthermore, VALVO (1971) noted in previously blind persons whose sight was restored by surgery, that the visual information was overwhelming, and the subjects often chose either darkness or a visual environment that was uncluttered. Further, MELZAK & BURNS (1964) had noted in their experiments with sensory deprived dogs that in the absence of prior experience, all stimuli in a new environment are equally meaningful or meaningless; failure to filter the information led to excessive arousal which interfered with mechanisms that would normally act in the selection of cues for adaptive responses.

The knowledge that plasticity does exist in the human central nervous system, as discussed in previous chapters and in other publications (e.g., BACH-Y-RITA, 1972, 1976b) should be sufficient encouragement to develop a series of new therapeutic procedures. However, objective evaluation is needed before they can be widely accepted. Objective evaluation has been particularly difficult to obtain in the field of brain rehabilitation. The long duration of the recovery, the absence of precise pre- or post-treatment morphological data, the plethora of empirical treatment approaches, are some of the reasons for this. LICHT (1975) has surveyed the history of stroke rehabilitation, which reveals that rational suggestions for physical therapy following movement disorders and stroke go back at least to Hippocrates and Caelius Aurelius. He discussed stroke rehabilitation programs in the 18th and 19th centuries that are defensible today, but which, up to World War II, rarely were practiced. They never received the attention nor the scientific evaluation necessary to attain medical acceptance. He pointed out that such an apparently simple problem as the absence of practical wheelchairs (until 1930) was a major barrier to patient rehabilitation.

Plateau learning

Patients are often kept in active rehabilitation programs until they have «plateaued», at which time no further progress is expected and they are discharged. It is important to note, however, that in normal learning of perceptual or motor skills, periods of no learning, or plateaus, are reached. BRYAN and HARTER (cited by ATTNEAVE, 1961) believed resumption of progress following a plateau is dependent on the organization of material into units, either perceptual or motor. Brain injured patients undergoing rehabilitation may similarly encounter plateaus, when no learning is apparent. If so, therapy should be discontinued, to avoid frustration of the patient and the rehabilitation team, but it should be resumed when the patient is ready to make further progress. This phenomena requires further study; maximum functional return may require several periods of intensive rehabilitation, and appropriate criteria will have to be developed to determine when the patient is ready for each step. In fact whether a corollary of FITTS' law (discussed above), or plateau learning, is more applicable to rehabilitation will have to be determined. It is possible that a combination of both occurs, with FITTS' law applicable to each step.

Neuropharmacology in rehabilitation

The use of drugs to aid in the rehabilitation process is not new. This field has been reviewed in Chapter 7. The possibility of their use in functional reorganization has been greatly aided by the demonstration that drugs do not have a uniform action on the brain; studies over the last 25 years (e.g., OLDS et al., 1956) have demonstrated action on specific brain structures by neurotropic drugs. Specific excitatory neurotransmitters and inhibitory transmitters, such as GABA, have been identified. A major advance has been the demonstration of the therapeutic action of L-Dopa in Parkinsonian patients. Dopamine (DA), a naturally occurring substance in man, was first recognized as the immediate precursor to norepinephrine and later noted to be an active substance in its own right. Dopamine is concentrated chiefly in the basal ganglia, but other regions including the hypothalamus and mesolimbic system contain high levels as well. Certain additional areas of the body lack significant DA stores but contain pharmacologically important DA receptors. These include the renal vasculature and a chemoreceptor trigger zone in the medulla. The discovery of DA's key role in basal ganglion function, which was confirmed clinically by the successful use of levodopa in the treatment of Parkinsonism, now stands as a hallmark of neuropharmacologic research (BIANCHINE et al., 1978). It is likely that, in the future, a number of drugs will be used in rehabilitation programs, the choice of the drug depending on the site and extent of injury. For example, many activities seem to require for their performance both a specific patterning and a general facilitation or rise in dynamic level. LASHLEY (1950) considered that the performance of any function is dependent on two variables in nervous activity: (a)

252

the reaction mechanism, and (b) facilitation. The reaction mechanism, whether of instinctive or of learned activity, is related to a definite pattern of integrated neurons whose threshold of excitability is variable. The availability of such a neuronal pattern, and the ease with which it can be activated, depends on less specific facilitatory effects. This theory of mass action or mass facilitation (LASHLEY, 1950) would appear correlated with the functional duality of the thalamus, in which the sensory relay nuclei have been considered necessary for signaling detailed information, while an «energizing» function has been ascribed to the generalized thalamocortical system (MOUNTCASTLE & POGGIO, 1968), although WALL (1970) has presented evidence of a wider role for the extra-lemniscal system. The reticular formation of the brainstem, and, particularly, those functional components grouped together as the reticular activating system, must also play an important role in the facilitation (see BACH-Y-RITA, 1972).

Drugs are likely to be available to increase general facilitation and to activate or inhibit specific structures or systems. BRODAL (1972) described the «enormous difficulty in initiating a movement,» while MINKOWSKI (1917) pointed out that paralysis seems to be a greater or lesser difficulty in initiating movements whose organization is undisturbed. A brain lesion may cause an imbalance in excitatory and inhibitory influences or a diminution of general facilitation by the loss of cortical tissue. In all of these cases, drugs with specific sites of action may be helpful in the future.

It is not necessary for a drug to have a long-term action to be useful. A drug with an effect of one hour would aid in developing motor control or sensory input during a therapy session, and even though the drug action did not last, carryover could be obtained from the experience and from the performance during the therapy session.

Age and time

The age of a patient who sustains a brain injury is a factor that affects rehabilitation (e.g., Chapter 1). For example, JEN-

NETT et al. (1975) have shown that «... age determines the possibility of good recovery after different degrees of coma; younger patients can withstand longer coma and still retain the capacity to recover.» However, although plasticity may diminish with age, it does not disappear. For example, the stroke case described by AGUILAR (1969) demonstrates plasticity present during the patient's rehabilitation from 65 to 70 years of age. Plasticity appears to be a characteristic of life up to the point of senescence (SCHEIBEL, 1978, BUELL & COLEMAN, 1979).

Time is certainly an important factor, in relation to the duration of therapy and the process of functional reorganization, and in relation to the delay between injury and the initiation of therapy. HARLOW (1953) found evidence of continuing recovery even in the last (sixth) year of his study of monkeys with brain injuries, and long-term recovery can be seen in man as well: LEVINE (1952) concluded from a study of the intellectual function of blinded soldiers that there is an «... amazing amount of recovery from intellectual loss occasioned by cortical lesions. Recovery from the effects of stationary lesions continues for a very long period of time and takes place for most and possibly all functions.» BLAKEMORE and FALCONER (1967) noted that patients with memory losses following excision of the dominant temporal lobe may show a remarkable degree of late (third to fourth year) recovery, and the stroke case described above revealed functional recovery continuing into the fifth year.

Functional reorganization can occur even when therapy has been delayed for a long time. However, improvement is greater when therapy is initiated early. BLACK et al. (1975) studied the contribution of active retraining to motor recovery following a standard lesion in the motor cortex in rhesus monkeys. When post-operative training in the weak limb was delayed four months, spontaneous recovery noted one week after the start of delayed training was about 50% compared with 9% recovery after one week in the groups retrained immediately after surgery (P < 0.001). The «immediate» groups, however, continued to improve over a six-month period to about 82% of their pre-operative performance. The

254

«delay» groups, by contrast, exhibited limited further improvement, reaching a plateau of 67% recovery six months after the start of retraining (10 months post-operatively). This difference in recovery between the immediate and delay groups was significant at the 0.05 level.

WEPMAN (cited by TEUBER, 1975) towards the end of World War II assigned half of his population of aphasic patients to immediate retraining while the others had to wait 6–12 months due to lack of facilities and personnel. The group that waited was subsequently trained as intensively as the first group, but at the end there was a year's difference between the two groups of patients on achievement tests in favor of those immediately started on treatment.

Motivation, environment, family and the mind-brain interaction

The importance of motivation in a successful rehabilitation program has frequently been noted and appears well-accepted. For example, HELD (1975, p.39) has stated, «We emphasize the importance of patient cooperation in his own rehabilitation. Patients who are apathetic, uninterested, unmotivated … show poorer results than patients who cooperate.» Similarly, a good environment, including good family support and good vocational prospects, are positive factors in recovery of function following brain lesion. Personal and cultural factors may also correlate with functional recovery. But *how* do these factors affect the neural structures responsible for the recovery? The studies of ROSENZWEIG and others (reviewed in Chapter 5) have determined beyond any doubt that the environment (enriched or impoverished) not only affects the structure of the developing brain, but affects the recovery from lesions. However, we are left without the knowledge of how these structural effects of environmental manipulation occur.

Rehabilitation as a specialty has a particularly difficult problem in determining its theoretical substructure. On the one hand, it must set its roots deep into biomedical theory (the principal reason for this book), backed by solid evidence. On the other hand, it shares with psychiatry, in particular, a need to examine and incorporate psychosocial factors, many of which have not been explained, and which may be unexplainable, by the biomedical model.

ENGEL (1977) has discussed the dilemma of psychiatry in this regard. He pointed out that most of medicine appears neat and tidy, with a firm base in the biological sciences, enormous technical resources, and a record of astonishing achievement in elucidating mechanisms of disease and devising new treatments. He considers that the problem of psychiatry (and much of the rest of medicine) stems from the logical inference that since «disease» is defined in terms of somatic parameters, physicians need not be concerned with psychosocial issues which lie outside medicine's responsibility and authority. He notes that «rational treatment», directed only at the biochemical abnormality, does not necessarily restore the patient to health, even in the face of documented correction or major alleviation of the abnormality. Conspicuously responsible for such discrepancies between correction of biological abnormalities and treatment outcome are psychological and social variables. He further notes that even with the application of rational therapies, the behavior of the physician and the relationship between patient and physician powerfully influence therapeutic outcome for better or worse, and that these constitute psychological effects which may directly modify the illness experience or indirectly affect underlying biochemical processes, the latter by virtue of interactions between psychophysiological reactions and biochemical processes implicated in the disease (ADER, cited by ENGEL, 1977).

ENGEL (1977) states that «... the physician's role is, and always has been, very much that of educator and psychotherapist. To know how to induce peace of mind in the patient and enhance his faith in the healing powers of his physician requires psychological knowledge and skills, not merely charisma. These too are outside the biomedical framework. ... It is the doctor's, not the patient's, responsibility to establish the nature of the problem and to decide whether or not it is best handled in a medical framework.»

The successes obtained with EMG sensory feedback therapy are probably due to general relaxation, to supplying accurate control information and to the active participation of the patient in his program. However, the success may in some measure be due to the confidence inspired in the patient and the attention directed to the patient and his disability by the therapist. It is possible, then, that a considerable portion of the therapeutic effects of rehabilitation techniques, such as EMG sensory feedback therapy, may be due to the mind-body interaction. The placebo effect is the best studied example in the medical field of the mind-body interaction. In a review article, Cousins (1977) pointed out that the fact that a placebo will have no physiological effect if the patient knows it is a placebo only confirms something about the capacity of the human body to transform hope into tangible and essential biochemical change; then, he states, «... the placebo is proof that there is no real separation between mind and body. Illness is always an interaction between both.» He further points out that in the absence of a strong relationship between doctor and patient, the use of placebos may have little point or prospect. In this sense, «... the doctor himself is the most powerful placebo of all» (Cousins, 1977).

A number of empirical techniques are used in the rehabilitation of brain-injured patients. In the hands of the proponents and their students, they appear to the casual observer to have considerable merit. But what is the basis of the therapeutic effect? Licht (1975) has discussed this question: «Soon after World War II, physicians and therapists announced schemes of treatment in hemiplegia based on neurophysiology both normal and abnormal. ... The practitioners of these methods are loyal followers of the principal proponents. ... Each (of the proponents) ... has written enthusiastically and seductively about their method. Each has referred to some venerable scientific names and studies. Each has attracted adherents who have unfurled and waved the banner of their sect amid ... many claims and counterclaims ... even though the number of rehabilitation centers which practice ... one of these methods is very small» (Licht, 1975, p.xii). He further noted, «The techniques of neuromuscular facilitation (one of those he referred to above) were taught to therapists (by demonstration) but often with a certain amount of the mystique which might be likened to religious ritual» (LICHT, 1975, p.18).

LICHT is certainly correct in expecting adequate documentation: «... if the proponent infers or proclaims its effectiveness, the claim should be documented with a controlled study, naming clinical findings at the beginning and at the end of a series of treatments, objectively» (LICHT, 1975, p.xii). However, it does not appear feasible to expect the proponents to conduct such studies. The proponents of these approaches are supremely confident that they are right. In my experience, in several cases, proponents of specific methodologies have said something to the effect: «I *know* it works. I don't have to prove it, since my patients are getting better. You prove it, if you wish.» The very personality traits that make these practitioners successful with patients (supreme, unquestioning confidence) make them poor candidates to carry out a scientific study. What percentage of their success is due to the specific methodology, and what percentage is due to the mind-body effect? A problem in carrying out a scientific evaluation with impartial therapists using the methodology is that this approach risks eliminating the mind-body effect, wich may be precisely the factor producing the major portion of the therapeutic response. Those of us who have been formed in the biomedical model find it disconcerting and even unpleasant to discuss the merits of the methodologies with the proponents, who totally reject the possibility that they may not be entirely correct. Yet their apparent success makes it imperative that appropriate experimental methodology be developed to study these rehabilitation methods. As the field of neurological rehabilitation develops more firm theoretical bases for therapeutic techniques undertaken within the medical model, it will become increasingly feasible to develop experimental methods to study the efficacy of those rehabilitation methods presently on the fringes of (or outside of) the medical model. Elucidation of the brain mechanisms underlying the mind-body interactions, and their role in the recovery from brain damage, offers the most fascinating challenge in rehabilitation research.

In summary, in this chapter some of the evidence for central nervous system plasticity was reviewed. The emphasis was on the scientific basis for the development of therapeutic procedures for brain injured patients. In addition, some inadequately studied, but potentially important areas were reviewed: these included the applications of neuropharmacology, the mind-body interaction, and the non-medical rehabilitation methods.

I acknowledge the helpful suggestions of Mark Rosenzweig, Ph.D. and Tecla A. Garcia, M.A., O.T.R.

Bibliography

ADKINS, R.J., MORSE, R. W., TOWE, A.L.: Control of somatosensory input by cerebral cortex. Science *153*, 1020–1022, 1966.

AGUILAR, M.J.: Recovery of motor function after unilateral infarction of the basis pontis. Amer. J. Phys. Med. *48*, 279–288, 1969.

ALBE-FESSARD, D., FESSARD, A.: Thalamic integrations and their consequences. Progr. Brain Res. *1*, 115–148, 1963.

ATTNEAVE, F.: In defense of homunculi. In: Rosenblith, W.A. (Ed.): Sensory Communication. M.I.T. Press, Cambridge, Mass. 1961, pp. 777–782.

BACH-Y-RITA, P.: Sensory plasticity: Applications to a vision substitution system. Acta neurol. scand. *43*, 417–426, 1967.

BACH-Y-RITA, P.: Neural substrates of sensory substitution. In: Klinke, R., Grüsser, O.J. (Eds.): Zeichenerkennung durch biologische und technische Systeme – Pattern Recognition in the Biological and Technical Systems. Springer, Berlin 1971, pp. 130–142.

BACH-Y-RITA, P.: Brain Mechanisms in Sensory Substitution. Academic Press, New York 1972, 192 pp.

BACH-Y-RITA, P.: Plastic brain mechanisms in sensory substitution. In: Zülch, K.J., Creutzfeldt, O., Galbraith, G.C. (Eds.): Cerebral Localization. Springer, Berlin 1975a, pp. 203–216.

BACH-Y-RITA, P.: Plasticity of the nervous system. In: Zülch, K.J., Creutzfeldt, O., Galbraith, G.C. (Eds.): Cerebral Localization. Springer, Berlin 1975b, pp. 313–327.

BACH-Y-RITA, P.: Brain plasticity demonstrated by sensory substitution and stroke studies. In: Austin, G.M. (Ed.): Contemporary Aspects of Cerebrovascular Disease. Professional Information Library, Dallas 1976a, pp. 87–93.

BACH-Y-RITA, P.: Comments on central nervous system plasticity. In: Proc. Second World Congress of the International Rehabilitation Medicine Association. Mexico 1976b, pp. 761–776.

BACH-Y-RITA, P.: Sensory substitution in rehabilitation. In: Illis, L.,

Sedgwick, M., Granville, H. (Eds.): Rehabilitation of the Neurological Patient. Blackwell Press, Oxford (in press).

BACH-Y-RITA, P., COLLINS, C.C., SAUNDERS, F., WHITE, B., SCADDEN, L.: Vision substitution by tactile image projection. Nature *221,* 963–964, 1969.

BALLIET, R., NAKAYAMA, K.: Training of voluntary torsion. Invest.Ophthal. and Vis.Sci. *17,* 303–314, 1978.

BETHE, A.: Plastizität und Zentrenlehre. Handb.Norm.Path.Physiol. *15* (II), 1175–1220, 1930.

BIANCHINE, J.R., SHAW, G.M., GREENWALD, J.E., DANDALIDES, S.M.: Clinical aspects of dopamine agonists and antagonists. Fed.Proc. *37,* 2434–2439, 1978.

BLACK, P., MARKOWITZ, R.S., CIANCI, S.N.: Recovery of motor function after lesions in motor cortex of monkey. In: Outcome of Severe Damage to the Central Nervous System. Elsevier, Amsterdam: CIBA Fndt., 1975, pp.65–83.

BLAKEMORE, C.B., FALCONER, M.A.: Long-term effects of anterior temporal lobectomy on certain cognitive functions. J.Neurol.Neurosurg. Psychiat. *30,* 364–367, 1967.

BLISS, T.V.P., BURNS, B.D., UTTLEY, A.M.: Factors affecting the conductively of pathways in the cerebral cortex. J.Physiol. *195,* 339–367, 1968.

BRODAL, A.: Self-observations and neuroanatomical considerations after a stroke. Brain *96,* 675–694, 1973.

BRUDNY, J., KOREIN, J., GRYNBAUM, B.B., BELANDRES, P.V., GIANUTSOS, J.G.: Helping hemiparetics to help themselves. JAMA *241,* 814–818, 1979.

BRUDNY, J., KOREIN, J., GRYNBAUM, B.B., FRIEDMANN, L.W., WEINSTEIN, S., SACHS-FRANKEL, G., BELANDRES, P.V.: EMG feedback therapy: Review of treatment of 114 patients. Arch.Phys.Med.Rehab. *57,* 55–61, 1976.

BUELL, S., COLEMAN, P.: Dendritic growth in aged human brain and failure of Growth in senile dementia science *206,* 854–856, 1979.

CHOW, K.L., STEWARD, D.L.: Reversal of structural and functional effects of long-term visual deprivation in cats. Exper.Neurol. *34,* 409–433, 1972.

CLARKE, E., O'MALLEY, C.D.: The Human Brain and Spinal Cord. University of Calif. Press, Berkeley 1968.

CLEMENTE, C.: Changes in afferent connections following brain injury. In: Austin, G.M. (Ed.): Contemporary Aspects of Cerebrovascular Disease. Professional Information Library, Dallas, Texas 1976, pp.60–93.

COLLINS, C.C., BACH-Y-RITA, P.: Transmission of pictorial information through the skin. Advan.Biol.Med.Phys. *14,* 285–315, 1973.

COTMAN, C.W. (Ed.): Neuronal Plasticity. Raven Press, New York 1978, 325 pp.

COUSINS, N.: The mysterious placebo: How mind helps medicine work. Saturday Review, Oct.1, 1977, pp.9–16.

CRACCO, R.Q.: The initial positive potential of the human scalp recorded somatosensory evoked response. Electroenceph.Clin.Neurophysiol. *32,* 623–629, 1972.

CRAGG, B.G.: Are there structural alterations in synapses related to functioning? Proc.Roy.Soc., Ser.B *171*, 319–323, 1968.

CREUTZFELDT, O.: Some problems of cortical organization in the light of ideas of the classical «Hirnpathologie» and of modern neurophysiology. In: Zülch, K.J., Creutzfeldt, O., Galbraith, G.C. (Eds.): Cerebral Localization. Springer, Berlin 1975, pp.217–226.

DASTUR, D.K.: Cutaneous nerves in leprosy – the relationship between histopathology and cutaneous sensitivity. Brain *78*, 615–633, 1955.

ENGEL, G.L.: The need for a new medical model: A challenge for biomedicine. Science *196*, 129–136, 1977.

FEINSOD, M., BACH-Y-RITA, P., MADEY, J.M.J.: Somatosensory evoked responses: Latency differences in blind and sighted persons. Brain Res. *60*, 219–223, 1973.

FINGER, S. (Ed.): Recovery From Brain Damage – Research and Theory. Plenum Press, New York 1978, 423 pp.

FITTS, P.M.: Perceptual-motor skill learning. In: Melton, A.W. (Ed.): Categories of Human Learning. Academic Press, New York 1964, pp.243–285.

GALAMBOS, R., NORTON, T.T., FROMMER, G.P.: Optic tract lesions sparing pattern vision in cats. Exper.Neurol. *18*, 8–25, 1967.

GRIFFITH, V.E.: A Stroke in the Family. Delacorte Press, New York 1970, 111 pp.

GUITTON, D.: The brain in our rapidly changing environment: Adaptable man? DRB Aviation Medical Research Unit Reports (No.DR 223), Volume IV, Dept. of National Defense, Ottawa, Canada, 1975, pp.252–264.

HARLOW, H.F.: Higher functions of the nervous system. Ann.Rev.Physiol. *15*, 493–514, 1953.

HELD, J.-P.: The natural history of stroke. In: Licht, S. (Ed.): Stroke and its Rehabilitation. Waverly Press, Baltimore 1975, pp.28–45.

JENNETT, B., TEASDALE, G., KNILL-JONES, R.: Prognosis after severe head injury. In: Outcome of Severe Damage to the Central Nervous System. Elsevier, Amsterdam: CIBA Fndt., 1975, pp.309–324.

KONORSKI, J.: The physiological approach to the problem of recent memory. In: Fessard, A. (Ed.): Brain Mechanisms and Learning. Balckwell, Oxford 1961, pp.115–132.

KOTTKE, F.J.: Neurophysiologic therapy for stroke. In: Licht, S. (Ed.): Stroke and its Rehabilitation. Waverly Press, Baltimore 1975, pp.255–324.

LASHLEY, K.S.: The mechanism of vision. XVI. The functioning of small remnants of the visual cortex. J.Comp.Neurol. *70*, 45–67, 1939.

LASHLEY, K.S.: In search of the engram. Symp.Soc.Exp.Biol. *4*, 454–482, 1950.

LEVINE, J.: Relative effects of occipital and peripheral blindness upon intellectual functions. Arch.Neurol.Psychiat. *67*, 310–314, 1952.

LEYTON, A.S.F., SHERRINGTON, C.S.: Observations on the excitable cortex of the chimpanzee, organgutan and gorilla. Quart.J.Exper.Physiol. *11*, 135–222, 1917.

LICHT, S.: Brief history of stroke and its rehabilitation. In: Licht, S. (Ed.): Stroke and its Rehabilitation. Waverly Press, Baltimore 1975.

LURIA, A.R.: Restoration of Function after Brain Injury. MacMillan Co., New York 1963, 277 pp.

LURIA, A.R.: Restoration of higher cortical function following local brain damage. In: Vinken, P.J., Bruyn, G.W. (Eds.): Handbook of Clinical Neurology, Vol.3, Chap.21. J.Wiley and Sons, Inc., New York 1969, pp.368–433.

MELVILL JONES, G., GONSHOR, A.: Goal-directed flexibility in the vestibulo-ocular relfex arc. In: Lennerstrand, G., Bach-y-Rita, P. (Eds.): Basic Mechanisms of Ocular Motility and Their Clinical Implications. Pergamon Press, Oxford 1975, pp.227–245.

MELZAK, R., BURNS, S.K.: Neuropsychological effects of early sensory restriction. In: Escobar, A. (Ed.): Feedback Systems Controlling Nervous Activity. Soc.Mex.Cienc.Fisiol., Mexico, D.F. 1964, pp.287–307.

MINKOWSKI, H.: Etude physiologique des circonvolutions rolandigues et pariétales. Schweiz.Arch.Neurol.Psychiat. 1, 389–459, 1917.

MOUNTCASTLE, V.B., POGGIO, G.F.: Structural organization and general physiology of thalamocortical systems. In: Mountcastle, V.B. (Ed.): Medical Physiology, Vol.II. C.V.Mosby Co., St.Louis 1968, pp.1315–1342.

MURATA, K., CRAMER, H., BACH-Y-RITA, P.: Neuronal convergence of noxious, acoustic and visual stimuli in the visual cortex of the cat. J.Neurophysiol. 28, 1223–1239, 1965.

OGDEN, R., FRANZ, S.I.: On cerebral motor control: The recovery from experimentally produced hemiplegia. Psychobiology 1, 33–50, 1917.

OLDS, J., KILLAM, K.F., BACH-Y-RITA, P.: Self-stimulation of the brain used as a screening method for tranquilizing drugs. Science 124, 265–266, 1956.

PAGNI, C.A.: Somatosensory evoked potentials in thalamus and cortex of man. Electroenceph.Clin.Neurophysiol. 23, Suppl.26:147–155, 1967.

ROBERTSON, A.D.J.: Anesthesia and receptive fields. Nature 205, 80, 1965.

SAUNDERS, F., HILL, W.A., EASLEY, T.: Development of a Plato-based curriculum for tactile speech recognition. J.Educat.Tech.Syst. 7, 19–27, 1978.

SCHEIBEL, A.B.: New insights into the process of aging in the brain. Brain Research Institute Bulletin, UCLA Los Angeles 1, 5–7, 1977.

STEIN, D.G., ROSEN, J.J., BUTTERS, N. (Eds.): Plasticity and Recovery of Function in the Central Nervous System. Academic Press, New York 1974, 516 pp.

TEUBER, H.-L.: Comment. In: Outcome of Severe Damage to the Central Nervous System. Elsevier, Amsterdam: CIBA Fndt., 1975, p.338.

VALVO, A.: Sight Restoration after Long-Term Blindness: The Problems and Behavior Patterns of Visual Rehabilitation. Amer.Found. for the Blind, New York 1971, 54 pp.

WALL, P.D.: The sensory and motor role of impulses travelling in the dorsal columns towards the cerebral cortex. Brain 93, 505–524, 1970.

WEISS, P.A., BROWN, P.: Electromyographic studies on recoordination of leg movements in poliomyelitis patients with transposed tendons. Proc. Soc.Exper.Biol. *48*, 284–287, 1941.

WHITE, B.W., SAUNDERS, F.A., SCADDEN, L., BACH-y-RITA, P., COLLINS, C.C.: Seeing with the skin. Percept. and Psychophys. *7*, 23–27, 1970.

ZÜLCH, K.J.: Otfrid Foerster – Physician and Naturalist. Springer, Berlin 1969, 96 pp.

Editor's concluding remarks

The contributors to this book have selected experimental results and theoretical concepts from the area of interest that they consider to be of particular importance for the development of scientifically based therapeutic procedures for brain damaged persons. Our goal was to provide a basis for others to design and test these, rather than to suggest specific procedures. We hope that each reader will have found information specifically applicable to his or her clinical needs. Although only time and future studies will tell which of the concepts selected are of importance for clinical rehabilitation, there are portions of each chapter that I consider to be of particular relevance:

Moore emphasized the need to consider the nervous system from a viewpoint somewhat different from that to which many of us are accustomed. She emphasized the hierarchial (archi-paleo-neo) organization and suggested that more rehabilitation emphasis be placed on the older systems. She would place more emphasis on the bilateral organization rather than the lateralization of the central nervous system. She noted that both sides of the organism are effected by a central nervous system lesion, which decreases the ability to relate to the three dimensional self and to the environment. She noted that the neocortical systems, which are crossed systems, are more vulnerable to lesion. Following a brain lesion the loss is reflected on both sides due to extensive interruptions of commisural fiber systems. The changes that occur on the «good side» are often not recognized when examining a brain damaged patient.

Moore presented supporting evidence for considering that the concept of the cephalo-caudal order of development should be re-stated to reflect the initial development of the cervical area, and thus she describes the cervicocephalo-caudal law of development. This, she suggests, should be reflected in the choice of rehabilitation procedures, with early emphasis being placed on the neck region. She makes a strong case for «forcing» the nervous system to use alternate systems when necessary.

Moore emphasized the importance of sensory systems in brain function. She then supported her contention that the classical long tracts in the spinal cord should be considered *integrative,* rather than merely sensory or motor. She noted that through vertibrate phylogeny the motor components undergo relatively minor changes, whereas the sensory systems show major changes and become of major importance. She noted that the motor systems are «servants» that can only respond or not respond, depending on the integrity of the sensory systems coupled with the integrative action of the nervous system.

Wall discussed the three major theories that relate to recovery of function following central nervous system damage:

1. Reversal of vascular changes and local tissue factors.
2. Sprouting of the remaining intact nerve fibers to occupy vacated synaptic sites, and
3. «Unmasking» of previously existing pathways, by modification of synaptic transmission.

He effectively dismissed the first as a basis for any recovery occurring weeks and months after the lesion; he noted the possibility that the second may play a role in recovery, but may also be maladaptive, and he made a strong case for «unmasking» as a mechanism of late recovery.

Glees' studies of hemispherectomy patients revealed an extraordinary capacity of the central nervous system to compensate for lesions, with one hemisphere being sufficient to sustain a person in locomotion, sensory perception of the whole body and a relatively normal social contact with the environment. Glees emphasized the bilaterality of each hemisphere as a major factor in the functional outcome following hemispherectomy. Glees reported that a study of the course of degenerating cortical fibers after small lesions revealed the plurisegmental connections of the major divisions of the motor cortex within the spinal cord. He considers that this most readily explains functional recovery following brain lesions. Glees discussed the possible neural pathways available to carry sensory information to the motor cortex, and emphasized the need for training the alternate pathways following brain damage.

Rosenzweig reviewed the considerable animal literature relating to recovery of function. Among the most important findings for the development of therapeutic procedures are the following:

1. An enriched environment (EC), which can loosely be compared to a therapy program, can compensate for certain brain lesions.
2. Two hours of EC per day is as effective as 24 hours of EC per day.
3. Socialization is not a substitute for EC.
4. Cortical lesions are not the only type of lesion that can be compensated for by EC; hippocompal lesion effects can also be compensated.
5. EC is effective in lesion compensation in adult as well as young rats.
6. If large brain lesions are made in several time-separated stages, the deficit is much less than if the lesion occurs in one operation.
7. In many brain-lesioned rat studies, there is secondary and progressive loss of cells, continuing over long periods of time. There is evidence that this occurs also in man. This suggested to Rosenzweig that recovery of function may be even more impressive than it appears, if it takes place against a background or progressive loss of brain cells.

Evarts noted the effect of basal ganglia lesions on internally generated movements, and the possibility of training compensatory external sensory guidance. Evarts summarized his extensive studies showing how motor cortex neurons participate in volitional fine movements. He described how the motor neurons relating to a particular movement are concentrated in a rather small cortical region (cortical focus), but the margins of this focus are not abrupt and there is a gradually diminishing fringe of neurons which can «take over» motor control when the focal area is damaged. He discussed the concept of «cortico-motoneuronal colony», a term referring to that collection of pyramidal tract neurons projecting mono-synaptically to a single spinal cord motoneuron, particularly in regard to the overlap of these colonies. He discussed the possibility that recovery of function following damage to a focus for a particular movement may involve the establish-ment of new connections from cortical areas which in the in-tact animal are in the recruitment fringe. Evarts discussed the role of the cerebellum in relation to its regulation of the rela-tions between input and output. He discussed evidence that the cerebellum plays a role in plasticity of the vestibulo-ocular reflex. Thus, there is evidence that the cerebellum may be of great importance in motor reorganizations which follow brain damage.

Brailowsky discussed the factors involved in drug effects, and reviewed the use of drugs to influence recovery following central nervous system lesions. Although neuropharmacolo-gy holds considerable promise of eventual importance in the recovery from such lesions, it is not yet important in the management of brain injured patients. Brailowsky's chapter provides the background for the study of potentially useful pharmacological agents.

I reviewed some of the clinical evidence (as well as several key animal studies) for brain plasticity. Personal studies were summarized showing that vision substitution is feasible in blind persons, and this was interpeted in terms of brain plas-ticity. The factors related to reorganization of function fol-lowing brain damage were reviewed. Two cases of excellent recovery from stroke were presented, one of which included an autopsy study. The factors and the neural mechanisms leading to the recovery were discussed. The role of the inten-sive home therapy programs which each of these patients had was evaluated. The mind-body interactions (e.g., motivation and the «placebo effect») were emphasized. The difficulty in obtaining the last 10–20% of recovery was noted. The extra effort required may make the difference between a handicap and a recovery.

One other factor, not discussed in this book, merits com-ment. No program, however well-founded scientifically, will be practical unless the costs are considered. Within several of the chapters are statements that may be relvant to developing cost-effective programs. For example, enriched environment studies (and studies of home programs, with family and community support) are relevant to group or community rehabilitation facilities in which the patient is in an environment conducive to self-generated and group activities, requiring less professional staff time. The importance of motivation and the mind-body interaction may lead to better methods (including neuropharmacological and psychological) of including these in rehabilitation programs. An increased knowledge of the specific mechanisms underlying the recovery process may lead to better rehabilitation candidate selection. An understanding of plateau learning may lead to appropriate use of intensive rehabilitation and intermediate care facilities. Patients could be discharged home or to an appropriate non-hospital facility during plateau phases and be readmitted when they show signs of entering an acquisition phase. This would reduce hospital and professional staff costs, decrease the frustration of the therapy staff and patients, and provide the non-hospital facilities (such as nursing homes) with a more dynamic image as partners in the rehabilitation process.

Lastly, a strong scientific foundation for rehabilitation medicine, in which all of the factors discussed here (and others as they are shown to be of importance) are appropriately studied and integrated into clinical procedures, is the best means of attracting the brightest, most motivated persons into careers in Rehabilitation.

Index